Real Beauty...
Real Women

A Workbook for Making the Best of Your Own Good Looks

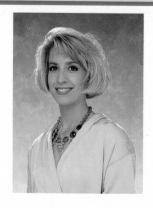 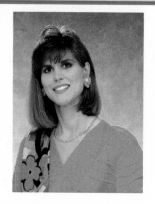 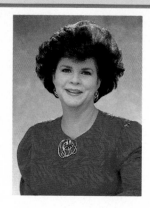 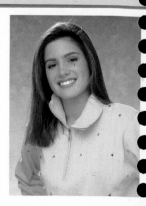

Real Beauty ... Real Women

Kathleen Walas

Library of Congress Cataloging-in-Publication Data

Walas, Kathleen.
     Real beauty—real women : a workbook for making the best of your own good looks / Kathleen Walas.
        p.   cm.
     Includes index.
     ISBN 0-942361-45-8 (paper)
     1. Beauty, Personal. I. Title.
     RA778.W16   1992   91-45412
     646. 7' 042—dc20   CIP

Designed by Antler & Baldwin, Inc.
Production services by Martin Cook Associates, Ltd.
Manufactured in the United States of America

10 9 8 7 6 5 4 3 2 1

This book is printed on recycled paper.

To Rick, Justan, and Alex...
your love is the real beauty in my life.

Acknowledgements

This book is based on information gathered over many years from hundreds of women all over the country. I thank them and am especially grateful to the thousands of Avon representatives who inspired this book and gave me insight into their own personal beauty needs.

A sincere thank you to Gail Blanke and Nancy Glaser who supported me throughout the process.

To Phyllis Schneider for her excellent research and contributions to the organization of the book, and to Beth Greenfeld for assistance with editing.

To Bob Antler who designed the book–a million thanks for your patience.

A round of applause for David Haney for his expert art direction and many long creative hours.

Special thanks to Linda Grimes, Kevin Luthern, and Rick Garcia whose makeup and hair talents resulted in beautiful makeovers.

To Jan Cobb and Marc Cohen for creating such beautiful photographs, and to David Croland for his outstanding illustrations and fresh ideas.

Thanks to Peggy Senatore for her fashion styling and ever-present smile.

Thank you to Susan Stautberg and the entire MasterMedia publishing team for their dedication and commitment to this book.

And a final note of appreciation to my colleagues at Avon who shared the daily pressures and office workload while this book was being developed.

Preface

Women's interests are similar in the areas of beauty and fashion—we all want to look our best in the least amount of time, with little financial investment. But learning how to put it all together can often be both a challenging and a frustrating experience. Where do I begin? Whom can I ask for advice? And do I trust their opinion on how to get it really right?

In an increasingly competitive world, we see that looking our best really does matter—especially in a workplace situation. It's certainly no secret that first impressions do count. More importantly, looking and feeling good for ourselves counts still more. Even in the worst of times, the better you look, the better you'll feel.

Yet, the "nineties" woman has been given a lot of options when it comes to improving her appearance. There are thousands of beauty products available and countless outlets for making her purchases. And the information available about what products to buy and how to use them can be overwhelming.

Over the years, I have "made up" and "dressed up" thousands of women across the country—from the woman next door to the star on the silver screen.

I must have had hundreds of those women say to me, "Can I take you home to do my makeup every day?" or "Do you have any suggestions about what kind of jewelry I should wear?" and "What hairstyle do you suggest for me?"

I wrote *Real Beauty . . . Real Women*, with the help of my friends at Avon, for the women of the nineties and beyond. The approach is simple and straightforward—a real workbook with space for notes; an opportunity to be hands-on in achieving your new look; a no-nonsense approach to the basics; an easy "how-to and why" format to help *all* women bring out their best.

Real Beauty . . . Real Women is not an exposé of the fantasy beauty of models or other celebrities. It

concentrates on approachable beauty for all women,
"making the best of your own good looks." I hope that
it will become your "live-in" makeup artist and image
consultant for the twenty-first century!

Kathleen Walas

Contents

Real Beauty . . .
Real Women

CHAPTER 1

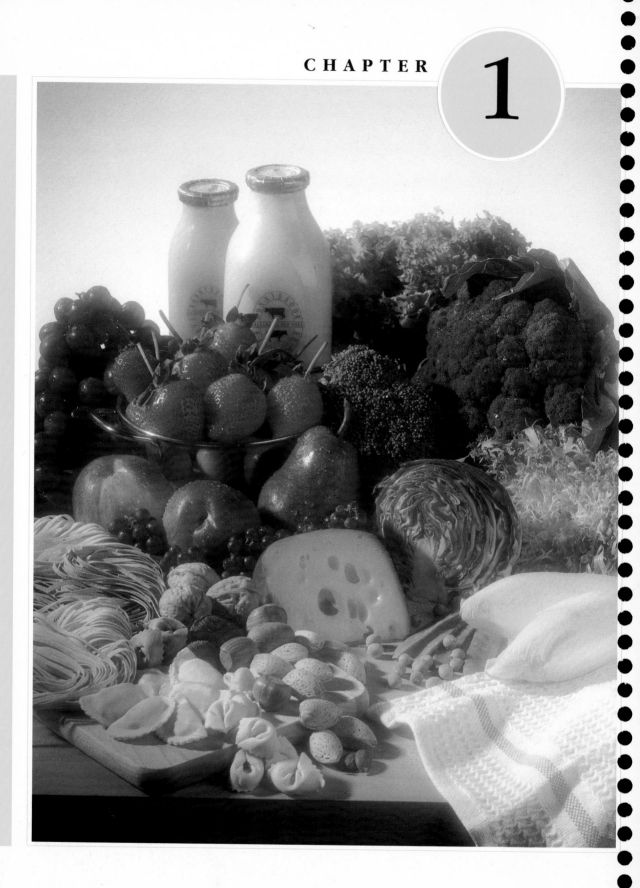

"Beauty" isn't merely a matter of appearance, of how you look. Rather, true beauty comes from a complex interplay of many things—the way you view yourself (and your world), how well you express your individuality, the steps you take to maximize your health and psychological well-being, and your ability to think *positively* (even when your world is topsy-turvy).

In the following chapters, you'll learn how to take control of your beauty regimen, with smart tips for keeping your hair luxurious, your skin radiant, your makeup glowing, your body beautiful. In *this* chapter, you'll see that you can take control of your life—and achieve a *special* beauty of *both* body and mind.

ACCENTUATE THE POSITIVE

Growing up, most of us were influenced by the media—and our peers—when it came to "looking good." Magazines and television shows portrayed the "ideal" woman, a gorgeous creature with model-perfect features, an impossibly slender body, a full, silky head of hair. It's only natural that we found ourselves trying to live up to that ideal (and patterning ourselves after our "prettier" friends, as well). But all too often, we may have developed the feeling that we just didn't measure up, that we weren't pretty enough—and some of us spent hours agonizing over our flaws—the too-heavy hips, the less-than-perfect skin—rather than focusing on our *assets*.

Lifestyle: Beyond Beauty

Psychologists emphasize that the way you view yourself can determine what you project to others. If you *feel* that you're too tall, for instance, you'll probably tend to slump a little, and others will pick up on it. But if you view yourself positively, if you truly believe that you're attractive, beautiful, you'll feel better about yourself in general and project that impression to friends and acquaintances.

Old habits (and beliefs) die hard, however, and

the woman who was convinced, as a teen, that her nose literally "took over" her face will tend to focus on that one feature for the rest of her life—unless she makes a concerted effort to accent the positive, instead of the negative. It *is* possible to change the way you visualize yourself by moving from a *subjective* to an *objective* point of view. Start by standing in front of a mirror and really "seeing" yourself for the first time. Look for your "beauty assets." Perhaps you have shiny, curly hair, or clear, glowing skin. You may have big, expressive eyes, or a smile that lights up your face. *Everyone* is special, beautiful, in some unique way.

Having a tough time being objective? Ask a good friend (choose someone who's fair: honest but not overly critical) to write a paragraph about the way she sees you. Have her list your strong points (your friend shouldn't limit herself to your *physical* attributes, however. Ask her to also note anything else she admires about you). It's likely you'll be surprised at the many beautiful things she sees in you!

Redefining the way you view yourself will take work. But as you begin to feel more comfortable with how you look (accepting your "flaws," celebrating your strengths), you'll find the result well worth the effort.

ON BECOMING AN OPTIMIST

It's important to carry the habit of "accentuating the positive" over into every other arena of your life. How you feel *inside* will show up on the *outside*, and if you feel happy, positive, in control, you'll radiate self-confidence and high self-esteem.

Some people seem born happy. Others have to work at developing an optimist's eye. Certain researchers feel that where a person lands on the optimism/pessimism scale is shaped during childhood by influential adults—especially parents and teachers. Others believe that your optimism level will change over the years—depending on what's happening in your life, on the type of people you work and socialize with, and on the ways you motivate yourself. If, on an optimism scale of 1 to 10 (with high positivity at the 10 spot), you find yourself stuck somewhere between 2 and 3, or

4

waffling between 4 and 7, is there any way you can move closer to the optimistic end of the scale?

Absolutely, say the experts. Here are ten steps for redirecting your thinking toward the positive:

1. Start by teaching yourself to view *problems* as *challenges* that offer you the opportunity to discover a creative solution and learn from your actions. Begin with smaller challenges: for example, if your ten-year-old's report card is full of more C-minus than B-plus grades, rather than chalking it up to "just one more thing I have to deal with!" view the report card as signaling an opportunity to sit down with your child to formulate a better study plan (and, perhaps, to spend more time with him), as well as prompting a meeting with his teacher so you and she can work together on your child's behalf.

2. Consciously set goals, at home, at work, in your community activities. If you feel shy about taking *risks*, start with small goals you're 90 percent sure you'll succeed at (for instance, acting as *one* of the coordinators of your church or temple's annual bake or rummage sale). As you reach each goal, set new ones. You'll find yourself striving to meet larger, more difficult challenges (and you'll experience increased self-confidence).

3. When you're faced with a big project (one you're not certain you can succeed at), break it down into steps, and concentrate on one step at a time. As you complete each step (or series of three or four small steps), reward yourself, increasing the value of the rewards as you go along. Perks might include a bottle of the new bath oil you've wanted, or a copy of a best-selling paperback, or a new skirt, or a pair of shoes. When your motivation really sags—or you start to fear you'll never successfully finish the project— promise yourself a special treat, a salon facial, theater tickets, or a weekend away as soon as you complete the job.

4. Anticipate success. Fantasize about what winning or succeeding at a particular task will feel, taste, and look like (do this several times a day, in the shower, on your way home from work, as you fall asleep). *Imaging*—or seeing yourself succeeding (whether it's delivering a speech to the PTA, putting together a presentation for your company's sales meeting, or speaking up on behalf of someone else)— is a very powerful tool. Olympic athletes, especially slalom skiers and divers, use imaging techniques to psych themselves for a win. For example, a skier fantasizes about winning in advance: she sees herself making a perfect run down the slope, easily negotiating all the tricky twists and turns.

5. Don't fight negative thoughts when they pop into your head. Instead, accept them, then *replace* them by moving on to the task at hand (suppressing negative thoughts only makes them resurface).

6. Surround yourself with successful, positive people. Success and optimism are contagious. So are pessimism and failure. You're doing yourself a disservice if you constantly hang out with people who have a negative attitude (that's *not* to say, however, that you should abandon friends who are going through a rough time—grieving over the loss of a loved one or worrying about possibly losing their job).

7. Keep a "win list" in your wallet or a desk drawer. On a 3"-by-5" card, jot down all the things you like about yourself (from your youthful complexion to your genuinely caring nature), *plus* the times you've succeeded with flying colors (winning the starring role in your high-school play, helping a friend through a difficult time, overcoming some sort of adversity, interviewing for—and landing—a terrific job). Go over the list every day (or, at the very least, when you're feeling down). By affirming your worth, you'll feel good about yourself.

8. Do for others. When your life is full of worries and unending tasks, you may feel overwhelmed. Take a moment and concentrate on cheering someone else up. Send an uplifting card to a sick friend; schedule an hour a week to teach an illiterate adult to read; work with a visiting pet program that transports dogs or cats to a local nursing home to cheer the patients; or volunteer to help cook and serve a meal to your community's homeless population once a month. Research shows that when you give to others, you tend to feel happier.

9. Try to read several pages of an inspiring book or

6

listen to a motivational tape daily (see a suggested reading list at the end of this chapter). A few positive words in the morning can boost your spirits for the rest of the day.

When life's really starting to get you down, rent an upbeat movie (a comedy—or a story about someone who's triumphed over considerable odds).

10. Do a periodic attitude check. During the afternoon, take five minutes to ask yourself, "How am I doing, feeling, today? Am I approaching this particular task positively or negatively?" If you're feeling angry, a little depressed, or just plain overwhelmed, try to get away for 10 or 20 minutes (if you're at the office, and are able to leave the building to get a cup of coffee, use that time to walk briskly around the block to cool down or regroup; at home, retreat to a relaxing bath, go for a jog, or just close your eyes, take a deep breath, and slowly count to 10).

STRESS BUSTERS AND ENERGY BOOSTERS

Stress can take a toll on your physical and mental well-being (lowering your immunity to colds, the flu—even to more serious illness, according to some experts). It can affect your sleep patterns, interfere with job performance, and leave you feeling irritable, drained of energy. Stress and anxiety can also show up outwardly, on your skin, triggering all sorts of disorders like psoriasis, eczema, acne, rosacea, and hives.

Here are some smart strategies for getting a handle on stress, and upping your energy:

Set aside "private time." A soothing soak in the tub (see the special bath recipes, pages 167-68) can renew you in mind and body. Ask your partner or a friend to watch the kids, then settle into a comfortably warm bath, scented with fragrant oils, for 15 to 20 minutes. Play relaxing music or meditate.

Learn a relaxation technique. Read a book about (or take a class in) meditation or yoga. Or find a quiet place (some people prefer the bathroom, where there are fewer interruptions), sit in a comfortable chair, with your feet on the floor, arms at your sides, and breathe in deeply. As you breathe out, repeat a "mantra," the sound "*ommmmmm,*" for instance, or "*mmmmmmmmmm*" or a meaningful word or phrase (recent research suggests that "prayerful" meditation—for example, repeating a line from a Psalm—heightens the relaxation experience for some people). Continue breathing in and out, slowly and deeply, and repeating your mantra for 10 to 30 minutes. If worrisome thoughts bother you, acknowledge them, but return to focusing on your breathing.

Do deep-breathing exercises several times daily. Recent studies show that by doing a deep-breathing exercise for just *60 seconds* five or six times a day, you can relieve stress and boost energy. Sit in a quiet place, with feet flat on the floor, arms at your sides. Breathe in deeply through your mouth, filling your lungs and diaphragm. Breathe out slowly through your nose. Continue, breathing in and out *through your nose.*

Schedule "worry time." Set aside 30 minutes each day to concentrate on everything that's bothering you (when worries crop up during the day, promise yourself you'll handle them during your "worry session"). End each session with a positive visualization or affirmation, imagining yourself successfully overcoming the "challenge."

Do aerobic exercise daily to boost endorphin levels (these are the "feel-good" chemicals produced by the brain). Evidence shows that a 25–30-minute aerobic workout can significantly reduce stress and tension, and up energy.

Follow a diet that includes "energy" foods as well as "calming ones." (See "Mood Foods," page 20)

Keep a journal, writing about things that are bothering you. New studies suggest that people who are able to write about their innermost feelings may enjoy better mental and physical health. Writing is also a powerful tool that helps you to organize overwhelming events and make them more manageable.

Eat a healthy diet. By getting the right amounts of carbohydrates, proteins, vitamins, and minerals (especially vitamins C and A, which are depleted during stressful times, and iron, a must for energy), you can not only keep your energy high, you'll also help minimize your risk of colds and flu. What's more, three

8

meals a day (with healthy between-meal snacks) will keep your blood sugar on an even keel, and you'll avoid the blahs, blues, and fatigue that can accompany a sudden dip in blood sugar.

Limit alcohol and caffeine intake. While a glass of wine may temporarily relax you, it can also leave you feeling lethargic. Caffeine *can* pack an early-morning and mid-afternoon punch, but limit intake to two cups of coffee, tea, or caffeinated soda a day. One cup of coffee in the morning can make you more mentally alert. Two can trigger restlessness and irritability. A cup of java in mid-afternoon can perk you up; any later in the day, it might keep you awake at night.

Cut back on sugar. Steer clear of sweets like cookies, doughnuts, pastries—they can make your blood sugar soar, then drop off suddenly, leaving you cranky, weak, unable to concentrate.

When you need an energy boost, take a whiff of muguet and peppermint. Preliminary studies suggest these fragrances can promote alertness. (See "The Science of Scent," page 199.)

If you're feeling tired take a 15-to-20-minute catnap. Studies show that short naps can energize you (don't doze for more than 20 minutes—you can wake up more tired than you were to begin with!).

Learn to set priorities—and say "no" to nonessential activities. Keep a calendar, listing all activities for a given week. Trim away those that are least important, or delegate them to others (for example, kids eight and up can help out by walking or feeding the dog, setting the table, doing dishes or light dusting, taking out the garbage). If a friend asks you to coordinate a community bake sale, and you're swamped with career or family responsibilities, tell her you simply couldn't "give your all" to the project—but ask her to keep you in mind for another project later on in the year.

Pamper yourself by engaging in a rewarding activity every day—be it painting, reading, gardening, playing tennis, swimming, or renting a movie you've looked forward to seeing. By focusing on an activity that makes you feel good, you'll not only boost your sense of self-esteem, you'll also begin to relax.

Laugh. Researchers have found that laughter is,

9

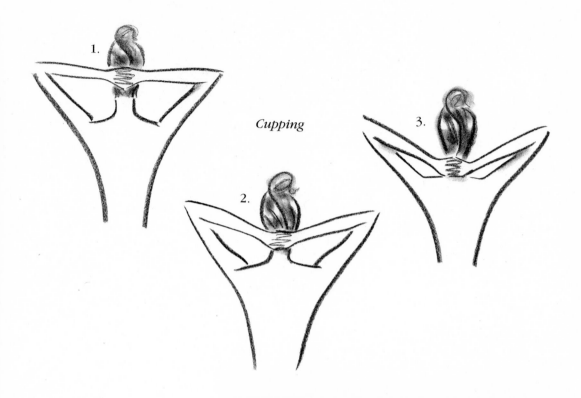

1.

Cupping

2.

3.

SOOTHING SELF-SHIATSU

In Japanese culture, bathing is an important form of relaxation, often followed by shiatsu, or Japanese pressure-point massage. Here, easy self-shiatsu techniques from Michele Schuman, a New York City shiatsu teacher and practitioner. (Sit upright in tub, or on a soft carpet or mat.)

Cupping. To reduce tension in the back of neck, interlace fingers and place cupped hands so that your thumbs are at the base of your skull. Slowly "cup" hands downward toward base of neck. As you cup, the heels of your hands should press gently on the long, thick muscles that run down your neck, about 1 inch from either side of the spine. Repeat exercise 4 times.

Shoulder Taps. To loosen "tight" shoulder muscles, relieve tenderness, use a loose fist to lightly tap along the top of each shoulder. Repeat 3 times on both shoulders.

Shoulder Squeezes. Place your right hand on the muscle inside your left shoulder blade. Using your fingertips, knead the muscle for 5 seconds. Repeat with left hand on right shoulder. Do 4 times.

10

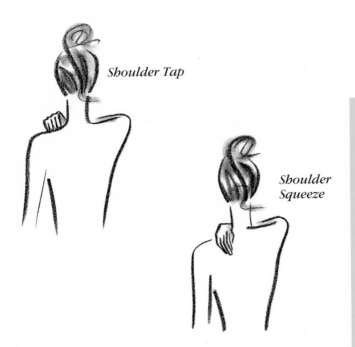

Shoulder Tap

Shoulder Squeeze

More Tension Relievers

·*Do 10 shoulder shrugs to relax tight neck and shoulder muscles.*

·*Alternating arms, reach upward, stretching toward the ceiling. Do 5 times, each arm.*

·*With each arm, do 5 sweeping circles.*

·*Do neck rolls. Let head drop forward and roll slowly to left, stopping just over left shoulder. Don't roll head backward (you can injure your neck); instead, move head to position over right shoulder, then slowly roll downward until chin almost touches chest. Repeat 4 times. Then, do 5 times, rolling head to right.*

·*If you have a sedentary job (sitting at a desk all day, or working at a word processor, computer, or typewriter), stand up once every hour, do above exercises, or walk around the office to relax muscles and rev up circulation.*

truly, the best medicine. By laughing, you increase your heart rate; stimulate circulation; exercise your diaphragm, abdominal wall, and other muscles; and increase production of certain hormones that serve as the body's natural painkillers. Laughter also provides psychological relief from tension, anxiety, anger, and emotional pain. To boost your laughter quotient, watch an especially side-splitting TV sitcom, rent a comedy, or read humorous stories or books on a regular basis.

Cry. The old saying "I feel better after a good cry" actually has scientific underpinnings. Studies show that the tears you produce when you're anxious, upset, sad, or angry contain "stress-relieving" hormones. (Conversely, those you shed when slicing an onion, or when a particle of mascara gets into and irritates your eye, *don't* contain these hormones.)

Treat yourself to Swedish or shiatsu (Japanese pressure-point) massage to reduce stress, unkink taut muscles, rev up energy. Massage helps release endorphins, triggering relaxation. (Or, do the easy self-shiatsu neck and shoulder exercises, see page 10.)

11

SLEEP LIKE A BABY

A good night's sleep is a must for physical and psychological health. Most of us need 8 hours of shut-eye a night. (Some people can get by on 5 or 6 hours; a few need 9 or 10.) A restful sleep allows your body to repair itself. If you get only a few hours of sleep or toss and turn, you can wake up with stiff muscles, dull skin, a lack of energy. Try these sleep-inducing tips:

· Go to bed and get up at the same time every day. By staying up too late or sleeping in—especially on weekends—you disrupt your sleep-cycle pattern and can prompt attacks of insomnia.

· A few hours before bedtime, relax in a comfortably warm bath. By increasing your core body temperature, you can gradually begin to feel drowsy.

· Exercise several hours before bedtime (to up body temp). *Don't* exercise right before retiring, though; you'll feel too energized to doze off!

· Avoid eating dinner after 7 or 8 PM. Digestion revs up your heart rate and can keep you awake. Try to eat your main evening meal four or five hours prior to bedtime.

· Do have a glass of warm milk at bedtime if you're feeling edgy. Milk contains the amino acid tryptophan, which promotes sleep.

· If you're hungry, opt for a *light* complex-carbohydrate snack. A whole-grain muffin or a slice of bread can calm you and make you feel drowsy.

· Stress can interfere with your sleep patterns, decreasing the level of serotonin—a body chemical that induces calmness. (Follow the tips in "Stress Busters and Energy Boosters" to relieve anxiety, pages 7-11.)

"In order to get the recommended daily allowances (RDAs) of most vitamins and minerals, a woman would have to consume a *minimum* of 2,000 calories, eating *only* fresh, nutrient-rich foods (that means no fast foods, canned products, candies, doughnuts, potato chips, etc.)," says New York City clinical nutritionist Shari Lieberman, Ph.D., author of *The Real Vitamin and Mineral Book*.

Even if you do take in 2,000 calories of "pure, unadulterated" food, you probably won't get enough calcium and magnesium, or meet your iron and vitamin B_6 needs, according to Lieberman, who adds that magnesium is as important as calcium when it comes to building and protecting bones; magnesium also guards against heart disease.

"What's more, the amount of minerals and vitamins you get in a nutritious 2,000-calorie diet may not be enough to protect you against the 'environmental insults'—the pollutants, chemicals, and UV rays—we're constantly bombarded with," notes Lieberman. "To protect yourself against these environmental dangers, you need adequate amounts of the 'antioxidants,' such as vitamins A, E and C and beta carotene."

Since most women consume substantially less than 2,000 calories per day (or get a major part of their calories from fats or sweets), Lieberman suggests that you consider taking a multivitamin supplement that includes a *mineral* component (many multivitamins *don't* include minerals). Or, you can pair a multi*vitamin* supplement with a multi*mineral* supplement.

Coffee drinkers should take vitamins in the evening because caffeine interferes with the body's absorption of vitamin C.

·Avoid alcoholic beverages. They can make you *feel* drowsy, but alcohol disrupts sleep patterns, and you may find yourself wide awake at 2 AM.

·Remember that caffeine can disturb sleep. Try to have your last cup of coffee, tea, or caffeinated soda before 5 PM. (Chocolate contains caffeine, too, and some people report sleepless nights after eating chocolate ice cream, cake, or candy, or

13

having a cup of cocoa.)

· Take a 10-to-20-minute nap during the day.

· If you find you simply can't fall asleep—or wake up in the middle of the night, mulling over a multitude of worries—don't lie in bed trying to doze off. You'll just become more tense. Get up, heat a cup of milk, watch TV, or read a book until you feel sleepy.

EATING SMART

Good health and *good* looks depend to a large degree on *good* nutrition. Nutritionists in the know advise that you boost energy, keep your blood sugar level on an even keel, ensure overall good health with a smart eating plan that includes daily choices from each of the four major food groups:

Dairy (milk, cheese, yogurt) supplies many nutrients, including calcium, riboflavin, protein. Requirements:

4 servings for ages 11 to 24
2 servings for adults 25+
4 servings for pregnant women
4 servings for breast-feeding women
(*Serving size:* 1 cup milk or yogurt, 1.5 ounces cheese.)

Protein (meat, poultry, fish, dried beans and peas) provides protein, niacin, iron, thiamine. Requirements:

2 servings all ages
3 servings for pregnant women
(*Serving size:* 2 to 3 ounces meat, poultry, or fish; 1 cup dried peas or beans.)

Fruits and Vegetables (juices, apples, oranges, bananas, grapefruit, melons, dried fruits, tomatoes, carrots, spinach, potatoes, etc.) supply vitamins A and C and some fiber. Requirements:

14

BREAKFAST OF CHAMPIONS

Experts agree that breakfast is *the* most important meal of the day. A nutritionally sound AM meal gets you off to a running start, helps you concentrate on mental activities all morning long, curbs your midmorning craving for sweets, helps prevent a pre-lunch energy drain.

Breakfast should provide you with approximately one-third of your daily nutritional requirements. To achieve this, eat one serving from each of the four basic food groups: for instance, a glass of orange juice; a bowl of cereal; a cup of milk (doubles as protein and dairy). Breakfast is also the ideal time to get your daily requirement of vitamin C and iron.

In a rush? There's always time for cereal or one of these power-packed morning treats:

· *Belgian Waffle:* Top a whole-grain toaster waffle with 1/2 cup part-skim ricotta cheese (sweeten with a pinch of sugar) and 1/3 cup thawed frozen or fresh strawberries, raspberries, or blueberries.

· *Strawberry Oatmeal:* Cook 1 packet instant oatmeal (for extra protein and calcium, substitute milk for water). Stir in 1 tablespoon strawberry fruit spread or jam before adding milk.

· *Fruit-Bran Shake:* In a blender, process 2 tablespoons oat bran cereal, 2 cups cut-up fresh fruit (bananas, peaches, berries, apples, or melon), 4 ice cubes, 1 cup skim milk or plain low-fat yogurt. Blend until smooth. (Makes 1 or 2 servings.)

2 to 4 servings of fruit for all ages
3 to 5 servings of vegetables for all ages
(*Serving size:* 1 medium-size whole fruit; 1/2 cup cut fruit; 3/4 cup juice. 1 cup leafy greens; 1/2 cup all other veggies.)

Grain (bread, pasta, cereal, whole-grain crackers, rice, bagel, muffin, roll, etc.) provides carbohydrates, thiamine, iron, niacin, some fiber. Requirements:

15

4–6 servings all ages
(*Serving size:* 1 slice of bread; 1/4 cup cereal; 1/2 cup cooked rice or pasta; 1/2 medium bagel or muffin.)

Most of us do eat adequate amounts of protein and grains, but many are likely to come up short in the fruit/veggie category. If you aren't able to include the daily requirements for fruit and vegetables in your diet, consider taking a multivitamin.

HIGH C

Your body doesn't store vitamin C, so you'll need to include C-rich foods (or juices) in your diet daily. (Vitamin C helps strengthen bones, teeth, and capillaries; there's also evidence that C inhibits the formation of certain cancer-causing substances in the body.)
Vitamin C also enhances iron absorption, so it's a good idea to combine foods rich in both iron and C at the same meal.

The recommended daily allowance (RDA) for vitamin C is 60 mg. The following juices are good, quick C sources (8-ounce servings):

Orange juice (fresh)	124 mg.
Cranberry juice cocktail (with added C)	108 mg.
Orange juice (concentrate)	97 mg.
Grapefruit juice (fresh)	94 mg.
Mixed vegetable juice (canned)	40 mg.
Tomato juice (canned)	33 mg.

Apple and grape juice are low on C—*unless* the vitamin is added. Whole fruits and veggies that provide C: oranges, grapefruit, cantaloupe, strawberries, green peppers, tomatoes.

CALCIUM COUNTS

Women need adequate amounts of calcium to

16

prevent osteoporosis (bone loss). When consuming calcium-rich foods, remember that caffeine can block calcium absorption, so it's best to delay your cup of caffeine until later in the day.

· Teens and women from 20 to 24 need 1,200 mg. of calcium daily.

· Adults, 25 and older, 800 mg.

· Pregnant and lactating women, 1,200 mg.

· Some experts recommend that women over 50 consume 1,200 to 1,500 mg. per day.

Calcium-rich foods:

8 ounces low-fat milk	300 mg.
Non-fat dry milk (1/4 cup dry)	377 mg.
8 ounces low-fat plain yogurt	414 mg.
1 ounce cheddar cheese	204 mg.
4 ounces creamed cottage cheese	68 mg.
1 ounce part-skim mozzarella cheese	183 mg.
1 cup frozen spinach, cooked	278 mg.
6 ounces calcium-enriched orange juice	225 mg.
3 ounces canned salmon with bones	203 mg.
3-1/4 ounces canned sardines with bones	351 mg.

To boost calcium intake, add non-fat dry milk to muffin, pancake, and waffle batters; hot cooked cereals; fruit "shakes."

UPPING YOUR IRON

Teens and menstruating women need 18 mg. of iron daily. Women who have gone through menopause require 10 mg. *Most* people consume only 6 to 12 mg. of iron every day. If you feel your iron intake isn't adequate, consider a vitamin/mineral supplement containing iron. Also, because caffeine can interfere with the body's ability to absorb iron, try to eliminate caffeinated drinks from your "iron rich" meals.

In general, the body absorbs iron from animal sources (meat, poultry, fish) better than iron from plant sources (dried fruits, such as raisins and prunes, leafy greens, dried peas and beans, potatoes). Iron-fortified cereals are a good option, providing about 18 mg. of iron in a 3/4 cup serving.

MORE FOOD FOR THOUGHT

· The United States Department of Agriculture (U.S.D.A.) recommends that sedentary women and older adults limit themselves to 1,600 calories per day. Teen girls and active women require approximately 2,200 calories.

· To protect against heart disease, limit your intake of saturated fats and cholesterol. Nutritionists recommend that you also limit your *total* fat intake (that includes polyunsaturated and monounsaturated as well as saturated fats) to less than 30 percent of your daily calories. On a 1,600-calorie diet, your fat limit would be

SNACKS THAT HELP YOU LOSE WEIGHT

Instead of . . .	*Treat yourself to . . .*
Chocolate milk shake	Chocolate float, made with diet soda, plus 1/2 cup chocolate flavor ice milk
1 cherry Danish	1/2 bagel with fruit spread
Hot fudge sundae	1/2 cup low-fat vanilla frozen yogurt, topped with 2 tablespoons chocolate syrup
1 small bag potato chips	2 cups plain popcorn (no butter)
3 ounces French fries	1 medium baked potato
1/4 cup sour cream (for baked potato)	1/4 cup low-fat plain yogurt
1 slice apple pie	1 medium baked apple (sweetened with fruit juice and sugar substitute)
1 slice yellow cake, frosted	1 slice angel food cake, topped with 1 tablespoon fruit spread

53 grams of total fat. On a 2,200-calorie diet, 73 grams per day. (Your best bet for counting fat grams in your favorite foods is a pocket-size fat-gram counter booklet, available at many book and grocery stores.)

· Have your cholesterol checked yearly (more often if you're at risk for heart disease). If your total cholesterol is above the 200 mark, you can help lower it by including soluble fiber, like oat bran, in your diet, according to researchers. Soluble fiber reduces the levels of low-density lipoprotein cholesterol (the type responsible for heart disease). Good sources: oatmeal, oat-bran cereals, low-fat oat-bran muffins.

THE SAVVY, SAFE WAY TO SHED POUNDS

Need to lose weight? Fitness experts advise that you combine *aerobic exercise* (30 minutes' worth, five times a week) with a smart eating plan that includes daily choices from the four major food groups (research shows that people who diet but don't exercise tend to lose weight less quickly and put weight back on more often than those who follow a sound diet *and* exercise program).

Cut back on fats (they're what really put pounds on!) and limit your intake of sweets. Weigh meat, poultry, and fish servings (2 to 3 ounces of one of these items, twice a day, provides sufficient protein for most women). Remove skin from chicken; choose red meats (and pork) with little or no "marbling." Increase your intake of complex carbohydrates (whole-grain breads, cereals, pastas); carbos fill you up fast, contain little or no fat, and your body has to work harder to convert excess carbohydrates into fat.

Unless you're on a physician-approved diet, don't dip below 1,200 calories a day; you'll starve your body, causing loss of *lean* tissue rather than fat. You'll also starve your skin—leaving it dry, dull, sallow. *Always consult your doctor before beginning any exercise or diet program.*

MOOD FOODS

According to emerging research, the foods you eat at breakfast and lunch *may* affect your energy level throughout the day. Some experts feel that high-protein foods can promote alertness (protein boosts your brain's production of dopamine and norepinephrine, the neurotransmitters that keep you alert, as well as controlling levels of serotonin, the hormone that induces relaxation).

· To up energy in the morning, combine high-protein foods, such as milk or yogurt, with a high-fiber carbohydrate food, such as a low-fat whole-grain muffin or cereal (the carbos will help you feel calm, more focused on whatever you're doing).

· Avoid gooey doughnuts or pastries as a midmorning pick-me-up. Instead, opt for a starchy/sweet snack like a whole-grain muffin topped with a teaspoon of jam. Carbos combined with limited amounts of sweets can restore mental energy. Or, snack on foods with high boron levels—pears, apples, oranges. Studies suggest that boron increases alertness.

· Steer clear of high-fat lunches, which can leave you feeling sluggish. Opt for broiled fish, skinless chicken, or tuna on whole-grain bread to give you energy for the afternoon.

· Studies show that caffeine *can* promote alertness; if your attention's lagging by 3 PM, a cup of coffee, along with a whole-grain muffin, can get you back on track (caffeine lifts you up, carbos keep you calm).

· Eat your lightest meal at dinner time. As the day progresses, your body metabolizes calories more slowly.

· Feeling especially edgy? Eat high-carbo foods like

A brisk 30-minute walk provides almost as much "calorie burn" and cardio-vascular-strengthening benefits as a fast-paced 20-minute jog, according to researchers. Use your office lunch hour or your toddler's play group time for walking.

whole-grain bread and muffins *alone* (without milk or protein) to relieve anxiety.

KEEPING FIT

Fitness pros recommend that you combine aerobic workouts with spot-toning exercises to keep your body trim (aerobic exercise also promotes cardiovascular health, as well as a rosy, glowing complexion).

·Exercise aerobically for at least 25 minutes, five times (or more) a week. Start each workout with gentle stretches to relax taut muscles and prevent injury to joints. End with a 5-minute cooldown.

·If you jog, choose running shoes that support your feet, keep ankles from turning. If you walk, opt for either running or walking shoes. Into aerobic dance? You'll need cushioned *aerobic* shoes to prevent damage to ankles, knees, and other joints. (If you take part in any exercise that

**GOOD READS
(FOR A SOUND MIND AND BODY)**

Balancing Acts! Juggling Love, Work, Family and Recreation by Susan Schiffer Stautberg and Marcia L. Worthing (MasterMedia)
Courage Is a Three-Letter Word by Walter Anderson (Fawcett)
Creative Visualization by Shakti Gawain (Bantam/New Age)
Living Happily Ever After: Thrive on Change, Triumph Over Adversity by Marsha Sinetar (Dell)
Minding the Body, Mending the Mind by Joan Borysenko, Ph.D. (Bantam/New Age)
Pathfinders by Gail Sheehy (Bantam)
Taking Control of Your Life: The Secrets of Successful Enterprising Women by Gail Blanke and Kathleen Walas (MasterMedia)
The Confidence Factor: How Self-Esteem Can Change Your Life by Judith Briles (MasterMedia)
Your Maximum Mind by Herbert Benson, M.D. (Avon)

21

causes your breasts to bounce, invest in a good, supportive sports bra.)

· Arthritis or other joint problems? Choose activities that place a minimum of weight on joints and muscles—swimming, brisk walking, stationary biking.

· To prevent exercise burnout, cross-train, doing one exercise one day, another the next, and a third the following day. For example, aerobic dance on Monday, biking on Tuesday, jogging on Wednesday.

· Can't leave the house to go for a jog or walk? Invest in a low-impact aerobics tape for your VCR (high-impact if you're in *very* good shape), a cross-country ski machine, a treadmill, or a stairclimber.

· Listen to your body. If you feel pain, stop exercising and give muscles and joints a chance to recoup.

BEAUTY WRAP-UP

1. View yourself as attractive, beautiful—and you'll project that impression to others.

2. Work at developing a positive attitude. You'll feel happier, more in control, and you'll radiate high self-esteem.

3. Start viewing problems as challenges that you can overcome and learn from.

4. Associate with positive, successful people. Optimism and success are contagious.

5. Alleviate stress with a relaxation technique such as meditation or yoga. Or, simply do a 60-second deep-breathing exercise five or six times a day.

6. Do aerobic exercise daily to relieve tension and boost energy.

7. Limit alcohol and caffeine intake. Alcohol can leave you feeling sluggish; too much caffeine can trigger restlessness, irritability.

8. Learn to set priorities, saying "no" to nonessential activities.

9. Eat healthfully, choosing foods from the four major groups: dairy, protein, fruit/vegetable, grain.

10. Avoid drastic weight-loss programs. Instead, combine aerobic exercise with a sound eating plan that limits fat intake.

11. Eat a nutritious breakfast to keep your energy level high, boost brain power.

12. Get adequate amounts of calcium to prevent bone loss, enough daily iron to prevent fatigue, anemia.

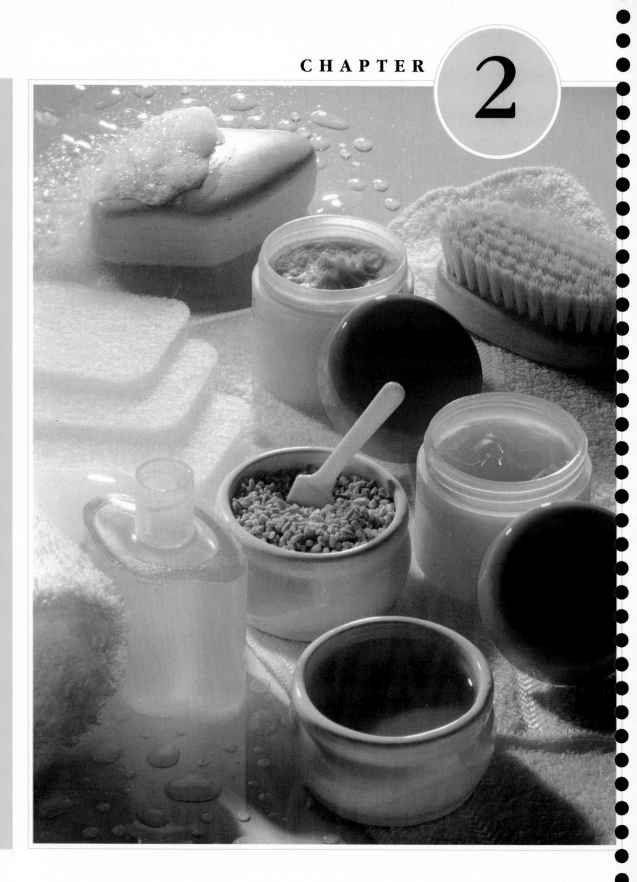

CHAPTER 2

Your complexion looks pretty good—right? Well . . . maybe it's a little dull, sometimes flaky. And you get a pimple now and then (or more often). Tiny red squiggles are cropping up around your nose and on your chin.

Stand in natural light and take a good close look in a mirror at your skin. Chances are, you'll notice all sorts of "baby blemishes"—like slightly uneven skin texture or tone, flat reddish dots or lines, an overall sallowness that hides your natural rosy glow. With every passing year, your skin shows signs of its age. But, thanks to skin-care products tailored to particular skin types and innovative new skin "treatments," your complexion can look healthy and radiant well into your sixties—and beyond.

SKIN TYPING

A good skin-care regimen begins with identifying your skin type, then choosing the cleansing, toning, moisturizing, and exfoliating products that are right for it. You can identify your complexion type by taking this 60-second quiz. Select the answers that best describe your skin, then jot down the number of each answer and total the numbers to determine your skin type

From Good Skin to *Great Skin*

1. How often do you experience blackheads or other facial blemishes?
   1. Frequently
   2. Occasionally in the T-zone (forehead, nose, chin area)
   3. Not too often
   4. Very rarely

2. How noticeable are your pores?
   1. Very obvious
   2. Very noticeable in the T-zone

25

3. Does your skin ever flake?
   1. Hardly ever
   2. Sometimes in the cheek area
   3. Occasionally
   4. Often

4. Is there a visible shine on your forehead, nose, or chin a few hours after cleansing?
   1. Most of the time
   2. Often in the T-zone
   3. Occasionally
   4. Very rarely

5. Does your skin ever feel tight or dry?
   1. Hardly ever
   2. Sometimes in the cheek area
   3. Occasionally
   4. Much of the time

If your total is:	Your skin type is:	Total
16–20	Dry	
10–15	Normal/Combination	
5–9	Oily	

CLEAN—BUT NOT "SQUEAKY"

Kind-to-skin cleansing is in. Vigorous rubbing and scrubbing are out, according to skin-care pros. The purpose of cleansing is to remove makeup, oil, perspiration, and environmental "grime" like soot, smoke, and dirt particles from the *surface* of your skin. Gentle cleansing will do the trick; scrubbing will merely irritate your skin, leave it red and flaky (overzealous washing with harsh cleansers—or even milder products that aren't right for your skin type—can make fine lines and wrinkles more noticeable!).

Cleansing is always a two-step process involving both a cleanser and a toner appropriate for your skin type. The following is a no-nonsense guide to coming clean:

Dry Skin has small, barely noticeable pores,

There are three basic skin types—dry, normal/combination, and oily. But, according to skin-care experts, your skin type can change or vary from season to season (and sometimes from week to week or day to day, due to hormonal fluctuations) and from climate to climate. Though you may *consider* your complexion *oily* all year 'round, it probably becomes drier, even a little flaky, in the winter, oilier in the summer. *Dry* skin can develop a hint of shine in the T-zone during the summer, while it's parched as a prune during the colder months. *Normal/combination* skin shows the greatest seasonal fluctuation—becoming oily during the summer, drier in the winter. Because of these seasonal switches, you may need to change your cleansing, toning, and moisturizing products two, even three times a year.

sometimes looks a bit "lackluster," and is prone to flaking during the fall and winter months. There's little or no visible oil on the skin's surface, and your complexion may feel drawn or "tight" after washing.

During the fall and winter cleanse in the morning and at bedtime, using a rich milky cleanser (usually a white liquid containing water, emollients, and soaps or mild detergents). Super-dry skin? Opt for a rinsable or tissue-off cleansing cream (always use toner to remove the last traces of tissue-off products). *In the spring and summer* switch to a lighter milky cleanser (not as thick or creamy as richer products), or a super-fatted or cream soap or moisturizing beauty bar (both contain extra emollients that moisturize the skin while effectively cleaning it). Opt for a very mild, alcohol-free toner or freshener.

Normal/Combination Skin is drier in the cheek area, oilier in the T-zone. *In fall and winter* cleanse twice daily, using a lightweight milky cleanser or mild non-soap cleansing bar.

During the spring and summer try a glycerin (transparent) soap to keep T-zone oil in check, while moisturizing the cheek area (glycerin is a humectant that attracts water to the skin). Use a mild toner to freshen skin in cooler months, an astringent to blot up T-zone oil during warmer seasons.

Oily Skin can look shiny or greasy within hours after cleansing. Often prone to breakouts, this skin type usually has visible pores and can look dull because oil buildup actually packs down flaky cells that have accumulated on the surface of the skin. *During the fall and winter* wash your face with a glycerin soap, an oil-balancing "soapless" soap, or a gel or foaming cleanser. *Come spring and summer,* switch to a mild soap formulated for oily skin. Use an astringent to sop up oil (look for one containing salicylic acid, which "sloughs" away dead-skin-cell buildup, while getting rid of grease). Use oil-blotting tissues several times daily to pat away shine.

"SOAP" VS. "SOAPLESS"

What's the difference between soaps—and soapless "soaps" or non-soap cleansers?

Soaps are a mix of alkali (mineral salts), animal and vegetable fats, and water. Great for removing dirt, bacteria, oil, perspiration, and makeup, plain soaps are too harsh for drier skins, but often work well for oily and some normal/combination complexions.

Super-fatted soaps are plain soaps containing extra oils or creams that counteract the alkaline—or drying—quality of the soap, and work well on drier skins.

Moisturizing beauty bars are soapless products that look and clean like soap, but they're actually made from synthetic detergents (very gentle—*not* like dish or laundry detergent!) plus special moisturizers. They're a good bet for drier complexions that are also soap sensitive.

Soapless "soaps" are synthetic detergent bars (and liquids) that clean skin gently and effectively. Often less drying than plain soap, many of these products are formulated for sensitive complexions.

If you live in a hard-water area, opt for a *soapless* cleanser, whatever your skin type. Soap ingredients can combine with the minerals in hard water to form a dulling, possibly irritating, and pore-clogging film on your face. Soapless products rinse away cleanly.

28

Sensitive Skin isn't a "type"—it's a "condition" that can affect any complexion, be it dry, normal/combination, or oily. Touchy skin is easily irritated by everything from certain cosmetic ingredients to very alkaline (drying) soaps. Look for mild cleansers that are free of fragrance, alcohol, and lanolin (three major skin sensitizers). If your skin reddens, feels itchy, or develops a rash whenever you use soap, switch to soapless cleansers, which are available in bar and liquid forms. Opt for cleansers formulated for sensitive skin.

Acne-Prone Complexions call for extra-gentle cleansing, according to Fredric Haberman, M.D., clinical instructor of dermatology at the Albert Einstein College of Medicine, New York City, and author of *The Doctor's Beauty Hotline*. "It's likely you'll be treating your acne with drying, potentially irritating medications," says Haberman, "and if you combine that with harsh or drying soaps, you can end up with rough, red, irritated skin." Instead, opt for very mild soaps or soapless cleansers—and don't *over*-wash your skin. Cleanse two or three times daily, and in between cleansings, use oil-blotting tissues to remove shine.

WASHING INSTRUCTIONS

·Avoid using too-warm or too-cold water to wet and rinse your skin. Temperature extremes can worsen dilated capillaries. Opt for lukewarm or tepid water.

·Splash skin with clean running water 10 to 20 times after washing to remove all cleanser residue. Left on the skin, cleansers can cause irritation, dull your complexion—even clog pores.

·Don't use deodorant soap on your face; it can leave a dulling, irritating film.

MOISTURIZER MUSTS

·While moisturizers don't actually *prevent* wrink-

29

From Good Skin to Great Skin

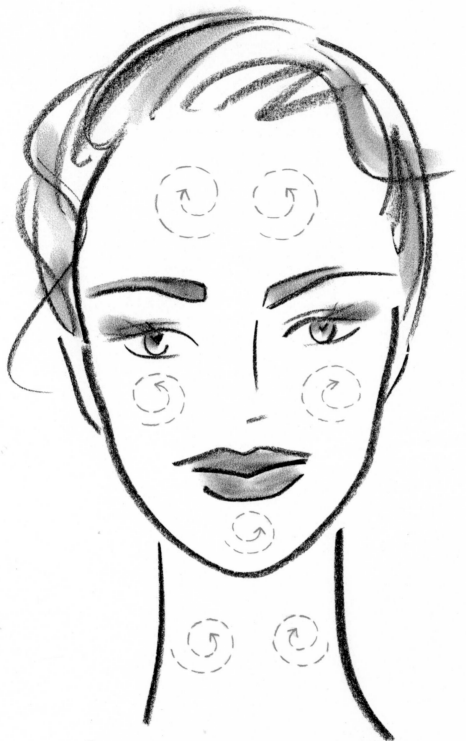

*Cleansers, toners, and moisturizers should be applied in an
upward and outward circular direction, beginning on the neck.*

les from forming, they *do* minimize fine lines (on cheeks, around the lips and eyes) by "plumping up" skin, giving it a smoother, more even texture.

· Moisturizers act as a "primer" for makeup, allowing it to go on evenly, stay put longer. Smooth moisturizer over your face and neck and allow to soak in for 1 to 2 minutes (applying upward and out toward hairline). Then, stroke on foundation.

· Moisturizers act as a barrier between the skin and the environment, buffering the skin against blustery winds, dry, overheated rooms, and pollutants like smog and soot.

MOISTURE *PLUS*

· Look for moisturizing treatments containing *glycolic acid*, which effectively penetrate deep into

---

DON'T FORGET . . .

· Massage cleansing product onto skin in small up-and-outward circular direction.

· Cleanse around your hairline and behind your ears. Shampoo, conditioner, and hair-styling products can seep onto these areas, triggering breakouts.

· Wash around under the jaw area.

· Finish the cleansing step by saturating a cotton ball with toner or astringent and wiping over skin (again working in an upward, circular motion).

Your skin's natural acid mantle (or pH level) protects it against germs, bacteria, and pollution. Washing can disturb natural pH, and it can take anywhere from 20 minutes to an hour for the acid mantle to re-establish itself. Toners and astringents tend to be slightly acidic—use them *immediately after* cleansing to restore your complexion's pH balance.

31

the skin to soften and renew even the driest of complexions.

·Opt for moisturizers with *liposomes*, microscopic "packages" that deliver moisture to the driest parts of your complexion.

·Choose products containing *hyaluronic acid*, which helps skin hold onto moisture.

MATCH MOISTURIZER TO SKIN TYPE

Dry Skin calls for twice-daily hydration (more often if your complexion's very parched). In the morning, use a rich lotion or cream formulated for dry complexions. At bedtime, replace the precious moisture your skin has lost during the day with a *nighttime* moisturizing cream. In warmer temperatures or during the summer months, switch to a lighter lotion moisturizer for day wear.

Normal/Combination Skin requires moisturizing in the morning and evening. Opt for a lightweight lotion product and apply to dry areas only. If your skin gets oilier during the summer, try an oil-free gel moisturizer.

Oily Skin needs moisture replenishment too—but only in the *dry* areas (the oily parts of your face provide enough lubrication to seal in H_2O). Use an oil-free gel-based product morning and night. Look for ones containing urea or glycerin; both are excellent humectants (compounds that attract water to the skin) and they're non-comedogenic (non–pore-clogging).

Acne-Prone Skin *may* need extra moisture. If you use drying medications like Retin-A or benzoyl peroxide, ask your doctor to recommend a flake-fighting product (in general, oil-free gel moisturizers containing urea are good bets). Women who take Accutane (the powerful oral acne medication that blocks oil production) usually need to use slightly richer moisturizers, like lightweight lotions, to replenish H_2O.

32

SKIN SOFTENING TIPS

· Does your moisturizer poop out halfway through the day? Fill a mister bottle with equal parts 99 percent aloe vera gel (available at drugstores) and distilled water. Shake well. Use to mist face several times daily.

· Use humidifiers in the living room, bedroom, and at your office—if possible—to add moisture to your environment and to your skin. Also, stock your home with plants that "exhale" moisture into the air—ferns, bamboo, coleus, spathyphyllum. Nix cactus plants—they *drink* H_2O!

· Tailor your moisturizer to the changing seasons (and to different climates when you travel). During the summer, add a drop or two of water to several drops of moisture cream or lotion. In the winter, mix a drop of chamomile or avocado oil into moisturizer to enrich it, advises Tamara Friedman, President of the Institute de Beauté, in Detroit, Michigan.

SKIN FITNESS

"Regular exfoliation is *essential* for a healthy, young-looking complexion," says Dr. Fredric Haberman. "When you exfoliate your skin properly, you slough away the dead skin cells that can clog pores, trigger breakouts, leave skin looking dull, sallow. You'll also 'uncover' pinker, healthier-looking skin."

"Scrubs" or cleansing grains, masks, even the common astringent ingredient salicylic acid, are superb exfoliants. (Some skin-care pros also recommend complexion brushes or complexion sponges for gently exfoliating dry or sensitive skin.)

Exfoliate once a week if your skin is normal to dry (dry skin builds up a dulling layer of skin cells quickly!); twice a week if you have oily skin. Sensitive skin? A super-gentle weekly exfoliation is okay (unless

From Good Skin to Great Skin

you have broken capillaries). Women with acne-prone skin should consult a dermatologist before using cleansing grains, but gentle *mask* exfoliants are generally a safe bet.

Choose finely milled cleansing grains incorporated into a creamy base. With the tips of your fingers, *lightly* work the grains over wet skin, using upward sweeps, then circles. Concentrate on each area of your face for a few seconds only. Exfoliated skin should look *slightly* pink—not red or irritated.

MARVELOUS MASKS

Masks are excellent exfoliants and can be used once or twice a week (in place of cleansing grains) to slough away dry-skin flakes, give the complexion a rosy appearance, and temporarily "tighten" pores. (A mask can quickly perk up "tired" skin, add glow before holiday parties!)

For dry skin choose a moisturizing mask (look for one that contains water and urea). *For oily and normal/combination complexions*, look for masks containing clay or kaolin (to soak up oil) or salicylic acid (to slough away dry skin flakes). *Acne-prone skin?* A clay-based mask or one containing salicylic acid or benzoyl peroxide (to prevent or dry up blemishes) is a good bet. *Sensitive skin* calls for gentle masks containing aloe vera gel or chamomile (both soothe skin).

You can also whip up skin-nourishing "natural" masks in your kitchen. In the next few pages, you'll find Ole Henriksen's favorite recipes. (Note: Before using any natural ingredient on your face, rub a "dime's worth" on your inner forearm and leave on for 24 hours to rule out skin sensitivity.)

MASK FOR OILY SKIN

In a small bowl, mix:
    2 ounces tomato juice
    2 ounces buttermilk

Cut three strips of cotton wool (available at drug-

34

stores)—a long broad piece for your forehead, a slightly wider piece for the center of your face (strip will stop at the tip of the nose), and a long piece to cover your chin and jawline.

Completely saturate each section in tomato/milk mixture; squeeze out excess. Lying with a towel under your head (to catch any drips), place strips on face; gently press them against skin to seal in ingredients. Relax for 15 to 30 minutes, then remove strips and rinse your face thoroughly.

Tomato juice is a gentle astringent that also normalizes the skin's acid mantle. It's also high in vitamins A and C, which are essential for healthy skin (see "Vitamin 'Therapy' for Your Skin," page 52). Buttermilk is a natural cleanser and oil-stabilizer.

HOMEMADE CARE

Looking for a gentle, *money-saving* exfoliant? Try this homemade "scrub," recommended by Dr. Haberman: Lather your favorite soap, beauty bar, or cleanser in the palms of your hands. Mix in 1/4 to 1 teaspoon salt (use the lesser amount for dry or sensitive skin). Gently massage over face. "The beauty of salt is that it dissolves in water," explains Haberman. "That way, you lessen your chances of *over*-exfoliating your skin."

Dry skin that's on the sensitive side? Los Angeles skin-care expert Ole Henriksen of Denmark suggests you smooth natural almond oil (available at health-food stores and some supermarkets) over skin before exfoliating. "The oil will serve as a cushion," he says.

Henriksen also recommends the following gentle oatmeal "scrub" for oily and normal/combination skin types: In a blender, shred 12 tablespoons uncooked oatmeal. Mix with 1/3 cup witch hazel and 2 heaping tablespoons plain yogurt. Store in refrigerator. Several times a week, smooth a thick paste onto skin and leave on for 2 minutes. Then, using a light touch, massage over skin. "Witch hazel blots up oil, yogurt cleans the skin, and oatmeal soothes and exfoliates," he notes.

MASK FOR NORMAL/COMBINATION SKIN

Mix together:
> 2 tablespoons honey
> 1 small banana, mashed

Cut a face-size piece of cheesecloth.

Smooth a thick "paste" of banana/honey mixture over skin. Moisten cheesecloth with warm water and place over face to keep mask from "slipping." Leave on for 15 to 30 minutes, then rinse skin well.

Bananas are high in essential fatty acids (EFAs), which moisturize and soften skin. Honey is a natural moisturizer that also creates a water-tight film on the face, allowing the skin to rehydrate itself.

DRY SKIN MASK

Combine:
> 1/2 avocado, mashed
> 1 tablespoon plain yogurt

Cut a face-size piece of cheesecloth.

Smooth mask over skin and cover face with cheesecloth to keep mask from slipping. Leave on for 15 to 30 minutes, then rinse skin well.

Avocados moisturize and soften dry skin. Yogurt cleans and soothes.

—Ole Henriksen

T.L.C. FOR LIPS

Your lips are constantly under attack—by sun, wind, chilly temps. Lip skin tends to dry out quickly, so moisturizing is a must.

· Don't lick your lips—you'll leave them parched and cracked.

· Do lock in moisture by using a lip balm, petroleum jelly, a dot of baby or mineral oil, or super-moisturizing lipstick every day.

· Lips are prone to "sunburn"—and ultraviolet rays can activate the virus that causes "fever blisters." UV rays can also age lips, causing fine wrinkling on and around the mouth. To protect against UV damage, use a lip balm with an SPF 15 sunscreen whenever you plan to spend time outdoors.

· Ski? Use a creamy SPF 15 lip balm—and smooth it on *generously*. Carry a tube in your parka pocket for hourly touch-ups.

QUICK SKIN FRESHENER

When your complexion's looking dull, tired, or appears red and slightly irritated (due, perhaps, to cold temperatures or too much time in the sun), revitalize it with this skin toner Ole Henriksen prescribes for his clients.

Mix:
      3 ounces strong chamomile tea
      3 ounces 99 percent aloe vera gel
      3 ounces witch hazel

Pour into a plastic container, shake well, and store in refrigerator for added cooling, astringent effect. Chamomile calms irritated skin, tones down redness. Aloe soothes skin, adds moisture. An effective but gentle astringent, witch hazel soaks up oil, makes pores look smaller.

EYE-DO'S

Next to the lip area, the skin around your eyes is the most delicate part of your face. Starting in your teens and twenties, protect this fragile skin from wrinkle-causing sun damage by wearing sunglasses whenever you're outdoors. Look for good-quality lenses that screen both UVA and UVB rays. For general wear, choose sunglasses that block 95 percent of UVB rays and 60 percent of UVA rays. For activities involving a great deal of glare or reflection (from water or snow, for example), opt for glasses that screen 99 percent of UVB and 60 percent of UVA rays.

37

To determine the UV-screening capacity of sunglasses, check the attached tag or sticker on lens.

More Eye-Saving Tips

· When you reach your late twenties or early thirties, you may notice a few fine lines beginning to show at the corners of your eyes. You can *prevent* these "crow's feet" by using an eye gel or cream containing sunscreen. Crow's feet already apparent? A moisturizing eye gel will "plump" up the lines, make skin look smoother.

· There are very few oil glands in the eye area, so *nightly* moisturizing is a must. Choose a rich eye cream if your skin is dry, a lighter one for oily and normal/combination complexions; smooth onto browbones, lids, around the corners of eyes, and over under-eye area. Don't *glop* eye cream on. Eye-area skin is extremely thin—and a *little* cream goes a long way (in fact, *too* much can result in puffy lids for some women). Don't rub creams into skin, either. You can stretch and damage this delicate area.

BLACK SKIN-CARE BASICS

Black skin is ultra-sensitive and prone to both hypopigmentation (light spots that can create a "splotchy" look) or hyperpigmentation (irritated skin that turns dark, creating a patchy, uneven look) and keloids, raised scar tissue that looks and feels like hard, dark bumps on the skin.

"Some women develop keloids very easily," notes Detroit skin-care pro Tamara Friedman. "Acne, cuts, scrapes, trauma to the skin—all can cause keloids," she explains. Friedman advises black women to "handle your skin gently—treat it like baby's skin.

"Hyperpigmentation can occur when you squeeze pimples or during a salon facial if the esthetician manipulates your skin too harshly (squeezing pores, for example)," she adds.

38

Resorcinol, a common ingredient in astringents and over-the-counter (o.t.c.) acne medications can also trigger hyperpigmentation, according to Dr. Fredric Haberman, who advises that rather than attempting to banish blemishes with o.t.c. remedies, black women consult a dermatologist. Physicians can prescribe topical and oral medications that will clear up skin problems *without* the risk of hyperpigmentation or scarring.

Other causes of hyperpigmentation? Electrolysis, depilatories, even plucking hairs. Overzealous exfoliation—with cleansing grains or roughly textured pads—can also trigger pigment changes. If you exfoliate, do it *very* gently and infrequently.

Black skin is also prone to "ashiness." Ashiness is actually *dry* skin, a layer of dead skin cells that give the complexion a gray appearance. Don't exfoliate ashy skin—you'll emphasize the problem. *Do* moisturize regularly, especially in cold weather, when ashiness tends to worsen. Also cut back on too-long, too-hot showers, which can dry your skin. Instead, take quick showers using lukewarm water, then slather moisturizer onto almost-wet skin.

EIGHT SMART FACE SAVERS

1. *Give your skin a daily workout.* Exercise increases blood flow to the skin—and blood bears oxygen and other nutrients vital to your complexion's health. For healthier, rosier skin, exercise aerobically three to five times a week or more for 20 to 30 minutes (try brisk walking, jogging, biking, aerobic dance—or work out on a cross-country ski machine).

2. *Steer clear of "no-fat" and extreme low-calorie diets.* You can starve your skin. For a healthy complexion, you need to include essential fatty acids (EFAs) in your diet daily; without them, your skin can become parched, cracked, scaly. A tablespoon of polyunsaturated oil (corn, sunflower, grapeseed) will help keep your skin soft.

If you dip below 1,200 calories per day, your skin can become dry, sallow. Eat smart, with choices from the four major food groups: dairy, meat, vegetables/fruits, grains/cereals.

39

3. *Sleep well.* Most people need eight hours of shut-eye a night so skin can renew and repair itself. Too little sleep? Your complexion will look dull and washed out.

4. *Stop to smell the roses.* Experts agree, stress and anxiety can aggravate—or even trigger—many inflammatory skin conditions, including acne, seborrhea, psoriasis, hives, and eczema. Turn to pages 7-11 for easy mind- and body-soothing how-to's.

5. *Never scrub your face vigorously* with a scratchy pad, rough washcloth, or harsh cleansing grains—you'll irritate your skin, leave it red and patchy (and, if you're prone to acne, you can aggravate the condition and trigger infections).

6. *Wash your face immediately after exercising,* or—at the very least—whisk away oil and perspiration with astringent pads. Oil and perspiration can combine to clog pores and to irritate the skin.

7. *Avoid wearing makeup when exercising.* Foundation can mingle with oil and perspiration to clog pores. If you'd like a *bit* of coverage, opt for a sheer, water-based foundation—whatever your complexion type.

8. *Don't open vitamin E capsules* and rub the contents on your skin or lips. You can end up with dermatitis (redness and itching) or a blistering rash. Do treat your skin to cosmetics (sunscreens, lip balms, eye gels, moisturizers) that contain E and other vitamins (see "Vitamin 'Therapy' for the Skin," page 52). Vitamins incorporated into quality cosmetics are so refined they won't adversely affect your complexion.

FIVE BIG BEAUTY MYTHS

Myth #1: Oily skin doesn't wrinkle as quickly as dry skin.

Truth: Oily and dry skins wrinkle at the same rate (how much and how soon you develop wrinkles depends on lifetime sun exposure plus genetics). Fine lines *are* more visible on dry skin, since the tight, flaky quality of parched complexions accentuates them. The lubricants in oily skin *camouflage* or "plump up" fine lines.

Many dermatologists do feel that women with oily skin tend to age a bit more nicely, however, since oily skin is thicker and its sebaceous (oil-producing) glands are longer and denser. These glands act like poles that run through the skin, giving it extra support, helping to prevent sagging.

Myth #2: Chocolate and fried foods cause acne.
Truth: Chocolate, French fries, fried chicken, and greasy hamburgers have been given a clean bill of health (on the acne front, at least). Some people *are* sensitive to certain foods and report that their acne worsens when they eat a particular item. If your skin breaks out whenever you eat chocolate (or another food), eliminate it from your diet for several weeks to see if your skin improves.

Myth #3: Even oily skin needs moisturizer.
Truth: Some oily complexions do tend to get flaky (especially in cold temperatures). A *touch* of non-comedogenic, oil-free mosturizer can help banish the flakes. But avoid putting moisturizer on oily areas (unless your doctor tells you to)—you can end up with a crop of pimples. Oily, acne-prone skin commonly develops seborrhea, a scaly, flaky condition that mimics dry skin. Many women (and some estheticians at skin-care salons) mistakenly treat seborrhea with moisturizers—worsening the problem. A dermatologist can diagnose seborrhea and prescribe medications that tame it quickly.

Myth #4: Astringents can shrink pores.
Truth: Astringents don't shrink pores. Cold water and ice treatments don't "close" pores. However, there *are* ways you can make your pores *look* smaller. According to Alex Znaiden, Director of Skincare Research and Development for Avon, "Many people are walking around with unnaturally enlarged pores." Pore size is genetic—you were born with a certain size of pore, and no cosmetic will "shrink" it past that size. But Znaiden notes that "a surprising number (60 to 70 percent) of people have pores that are enlarged because they're clogged with oil, cellular debris, and dirt. If you clean out the pores, you can get them back to the size

41

they're supposed to be." In this sense, pores *can* be made smaller.

Pore "reducing" masks (especially those containing salicylic acid and benzoyl peroxide), cleansing grains, astringents (containing salicylic acid or resorcinol) can slough away the dry, flaky skin that clogs pores and impedes proper oil flow.

More pore "tighteners"? Most astringents slightly irritate the skin, plumping it up around pores to make them appear smaller. Because oil can pool in pores, giving them a darker appearance, you'll want to remove the grease with astringents, cleansers, or oil-blotting tissues.

Products containing retinol (vitamin A) are believed to reduce the size of pores by normalizing and reducing the amount of sebum produced by the sebaceous glands.

Myth #5: The sun will clear up acne.

Truth: A tan temporarily camouflages blemishes, but heat, humidity, and UV rays can aggravate acne by

42

overstimulating the oil glands. What's more, a tan "thickens" the outer layer of the skin—blocking pores. Come fall, when your tan begins to fade, you may find a crop of post-summer pimples (dermatologists report that acne cases surge in September and October).

"UV light also produces free radicals, which cause changes to occur in the quality of sebum. Natural, free-flowing sebum can be transformed into waxy materials that are difficult to get out of pores. This can lead to clogged pores and blemishes," says Alex Znaiden.

BEAUTY WRAP-UP

1. Your skin type can vary with the seasons. Change your complexion-care products accordingly, opting for lighter cleansers, toners, and moisturizers during the summer, richer ones in the winter.

2. If your skin gets red, rashy, or itchy whenever you use soap, switch to a soapless cleanser. If you live in a hard-water area, choose soapless products; soap can combine with the minerals in hard water to form a complexion-dulling, pore-clogging film on your skin. Soap-free products rinse cleanly away.

3. Don't forget to cleanse the "hidden" areas—around your hairline, behind your ears, under your jaw. Saturate a cotton ball with astringent or toner and whisk over skin to clean.

4. Use moisturizer to "plump up" fine wrinkles—and to act as a protective barrier between your skin and the environment.

5. Exfoliate your skin regularly to remove the dry, flaky patches that can clog pores, dull your complexion.

6. If you have black skin, prevent ashiness by moisturizing skin frequently.

7. Exercise aerobically every day to keep your skin "fit," rosy-looking.

CHAPTER

3

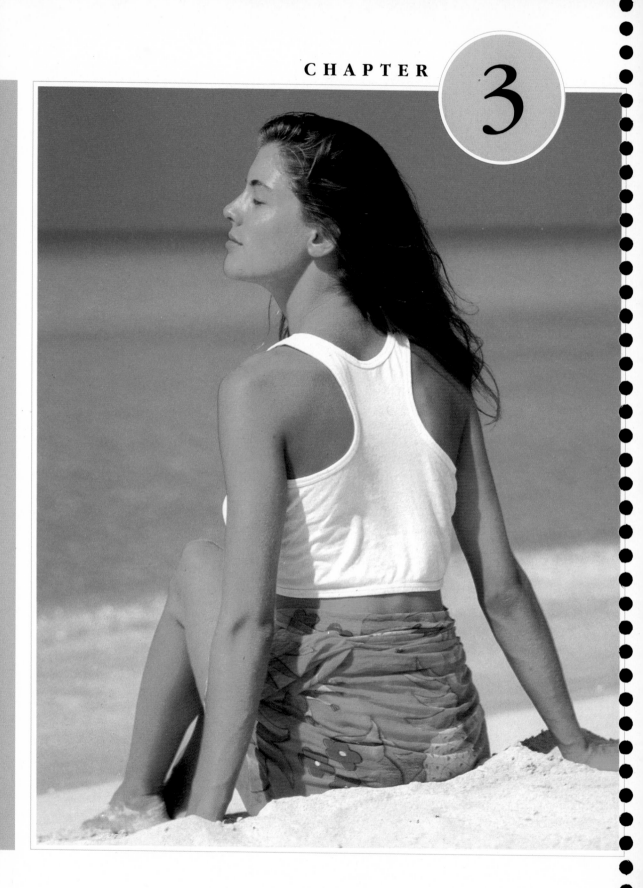

"Between 50 and 60 percent of my *adult* patients come to me for acne treatment," says dermatologist Fredric Haberman. According to Dr. Haberman and other experts, more and more women are experiencing breakouts in their twenties, thirties, and forties, and even in their fifties and sixties. While hormonal fluctuations (due to menstruation, childbirth, and menopause) account for many cases, Haberman notes that *stress*—the pressures of juggling families and careers—can wreak havoc with adult skin. "Stress triggers surges of various acne-triggering hormones," he explains. While treating patients with oral and topical medications, he also advises them to "slow down, relax." (See "Stress Busters," page 7-11.)

Adolescent acne—the kind you had as a teenager—can come back with a vengeance in your later years. Some women, who never had a pimple during their teen years, find they're suddenly breaking out in their thirties. Very mild cases of acne (the scientific name is "acne vulgaris") can be treated with over-the-counter products. Moderate to severe cases require treatment by a dermatologist, who can prescribe topical and/or oral medications to control the eruptions. Left untreated, acne *can* cause permanent scarring.

Skin Spoilers

Just an occasional pimple, blackhead, or whitehead? Opt for benzoyl peroxide lotions or creams (available over-the-counter in 2.5, 5, and 10 percent strengths) to dry up pimples, prevent new ones from forming—and to "root out" blackheads. Or, speed healing of existing pimples (and prevent new ones from forming) with medications containing salicylic acid or resorcinol—both slough away dead skin cells that clog pores.

Always wait 30 minutes after cleansing your face before applying benzoyl peroxide. Smoothed onto just-washed skin, it can cause irritation, redness, peeling (for that matter, so can the prescription acne medication Retin-A).

Acne rosacea (also called "adult acne") is a common condition that can appear as early as the twenties, but is more likely to surface in the thirties or forties. Researchers believe certain people are genetically predisposed to developing rosacea, which is characterized by numerous tiny dilated blood vessels on and around the nose, cheeks, and chin, and in some cases by little red bumps and large, inflamed acne-like cysts.

Stress can trigger a rosacea flare-up. So can very hot and very cold beverages, alcoholic drinks, caffeine, spicy foods, super-hot temperatures, and blasts of heat—from a conventional oven or toaster oven. Certain infections and some dental procedures can also aggravate rosacea.

Moderate to severe rosacea cases should be treated by a dermatologist, who can prescribe topical (and, sometimes, oral) antibiotics, sulfur creams, and hydrocortisone lotions. For very mild cases, try these skin-soothers to "take the red out":

· Soak big cotton puffs or strips in cooled chamomile tea. Squeeze out excess moisture, then pat over red areas.

· Soak a clean washcloth in cool milk. Wring out and place on face for 5 minutes.

Don't *over*-cleanse rosacea-prone skin. You can irritate it. Also, avoid skin "massage" or salon facials that include squeezing pores, which can increase the likelihood of dilated capillaries.

Acne cosmetica is another skin problem plaguing many women. Certain ingredients in cosmetics can clog pores, trigger breakouts (that's why it's important to look for cleansers and makeups labeled "non-comedogenic" or "non-acnegenic" if you're prone to blackheads and pimples). Combinations of certain cosmetics can also lead to blocked pores and eruptions. Even a woman who has extremely *dry* skin can break out if she uses a heavy, creamy cleanser, a heavy moisturizer, *and* a thick, pore-clogging foundation.

Cosmetic-related acne can show up on your face within 24 hours after using a particular product—or it may take weeks to develop. "Isolating the offending in-

46

BLEMISH BANISHERS

· Stop a pimple from forming (and minimize redness) by placing two crushed ice cubes in a plastic sandwich bag and holding it against the blemish for 3 minutes, several times a day. Apply benzoyl peroxide immediately after each "ice treatment."

· Wake up with a *big* red bump—or an unsightly white-capped pimple that concealer won't hide? Don't prick open the cap. You can cause further infection, possible scarring. Instead, help deflate the pimple and lessen the redness by steaming clean skin for 5 minutes: Boil 4 pints of water and pour into a large bowl. Drape a towel over your head, and bend over the bowl (don't get too close). Then saturate a cotton ball with *very warm* salt water (mix 1 teaspoon salt into 1 pint water). Hold cotton against pimple for 2 to 5 minutes (repeat treatment during the day). Eventually, the cap will disappear into the blemish.

· Don't use foundation or concealer on an "open" pimple—one whose white cap has been dislodged. Instead, dot on a minimal amount of tinted acne medication to conceal.

gredient or cosmetic is difficult," says Haberman, who advises that if you suspect your breakouts are triggered by cosmetics, you "pack up all your beauty aids, from cleansers to foundations to hair preparations, and take them to your dermatologist. He or she may be able to find the culprit."

Chemical acne affects people who are sensitive to iodine or bromides, and most commonly appears around the mouth as blackheads, whiteheads, or little red pimples—but occasionally can occur on other areas of the face (and back and chest) in what look like big, inflamed acne cysts. Chemical acne can crop up within 12 to 24 hours after you've eaten food high in iodine (shellfish, beef liver, canned or frozen food high in iodized salt) or taken medications or vitamins taining iodine or bromides (some cough medicines, and vitamins containing kelp or seaweed).

You can speed healing of minor blemishes by using a benzoyl peroxide cream twice a day. Larger cysts can linger for weeks (and may cause scarring). A dermatologist can inject them with a weak corticosteroid solution so they'll "deflate" within 24 hours.

SKIN PERFECTERS

Q. Can dilated capillaries on the face be removed?
A. A qualified dermatologist or plastic surgeon can seal these little vessels, stopping the flow of blood, with in-office electrosurgery, using a fine electric-current needle and very low wattage. More stubborn vessels may require low-current laser treatment.

In the near future a patented, breakthrough topical preparation will be marketed that will eliminate dilated capillaries, averting the need to see a dermatologist or plastic surgeon.

Q. Can brownish "age" spots be lightened or removed?
A. A dermatologist can use liquid nitrogen to freeze and remove age spots. Light facial peels using trichloroacetic acid (TCA) can minimize some spots, and over-the-counter bleaching creams containing hydroquinone, resorcinol, or salicylic acid can be used at home. (You'll need to repeat the "bleaching treatment" several times for best results.) Some studies show that long-term use of topical trentinoin, vitamin A acid, and glycolic acid products can lighten or even eliminate age spots.

DE-FUZZERS

Lots of hair on your head is a beauty plus. Hair on your face isn't. Use one of the following methods to get rid of—or camouflage—unwanted facial hair.

Bleaching is a good bet if you want to lighten hair on your upper lip. *Be sure to choose a product formulated for use on facial skin. Pros:* Bleaching is easy and inexpensive, and works well on a light growth of light-to-medium-brown hair. *Cons:* Can turn dark-brown hair orangey. May irritate skin (especially sensitive complexions and over-forty skin, which tends to be drier, more prone to irritation). Always do a 24-hour patch test on your inner forearm before using bleach on your face.

Tweezing is an effective way of removing isolated hairs around the outer corners of the mouth and on the chin. Opt for fine-point tweezers that firmly grip hairs. Cleanse skin with a mild lotion before tweezing, and pat on a gentle astringent and light moisturizer afterward. *Pros:* Fast, easy, inexpensive. *Cons:* Can be painful—and skin may become irritated.

Depilatories dissolve hair just above the skin line and can be used to remove upper-lip fuzz *(look for a product formulated for facial skin)*. *Pros:* Easy and inexpensive, leaving skin super-smooth. *Cons:* Can trigger redness, irritation. (Do a skin-patch test each time you use a depilatory; sensitivity can develop after weeks—or even months—of using a particular product.) Minimize the chance of irritation by choosing products containing aloe or mineral oil. Apply a small amount of petroleum jelly on upper lip after removing cream. Avoid cosmetics or rich moisturizers for 3 to 5 hours afterward. Wait 24 hours before sunning or swimming in a chlorinated pool.

Waxing removes hairs slightly below the surface of the skin and is ideal for getting rid of a mustache. In "hot" waxing, heated then slightly cooled wax is applied to the skin, left to dry, then peeled off—taking the hair and a bit of root with it. In "cold" waxing, a putty-like substance is pressed onto the skin, then quickly pulled off. *Pros:* Results can last for six to eight weeks. *Cons:* May be painful, can cause ingrown hairs. A two-to-three-week growth of hair is required for best results. Rely on a skilled esthetician for hot waxing. You can use a cold wax product at home—but follow instructions carefully.

Electrolysis uses electrical current to destroy the hair follicle, making it unable to produce more hairs. Can be used on the upper lip and chin. *Pros:* Hair removal is permanent. *Cons:* Can be painful (especially in lip area), expensive, and time-consuming (you'll need several months of treatments to remove all the hair on your upper lip). May cause temporary redness or scabbing. Improperly done, electrolysis can cause scarring, worsen dilated capillaries. *Ask a dermatologist or esthetician to recommend a qualified, highly skilled electrologist.*

THE SKIN "AGERS"

(Tracking down the *real* causes of wrinkles, "age" spots, patchy skin, and other little uglies.)

Your skin ages from the inside (intrinsically) and the outside (extrinsically). Natural or intrinsic aging, caused by heredity and passing years, doesn't show up on your face until your late fifties or early sixties, when fine and deeper wrinkles, thinning skin, and a loss of elasticity become more apparent.

Extrinsic aging, triggered by outside factors, worsen with every passing decade.

Here, the four most common causes of extrinsic aging (and how you can prevent or reverse their effects on your skin):

1. *Sun exposure* is, according to experts, responsible for up to 90 percent of fine and deep wrinkling (heredity and chronological age account for only about 10 percent!). What's more, photoaging (damage to the skin by the sun's ultraviolet—or UV—rays) is also to blame for the flat brown "age" spots that appear on the face, hands, and arms; rough, uneven textured skin; uneven skin tone; dilated or "broken" capillaries; and an overall dullness or "yellowing" of the skin.

2. *Expression lines* (furrows across your forehead, "laugh lines" that run from the sides of your nostrils to the corners of your mouth, "crinkles" around the eyes) are caused in part by repeated facial expressions such as smiling, frowning, and squinting. Hints of these lines appear in the twenties, are a permanent part of your face by the thirties and forties. (Note: Despite what you may have heard, "facial exercises" don't promote skin health. Avoid these "grimace" and "scrunch" exercises, which can actually deepen expression lines.)

3. *Sleep lines* are the result of pushing or burrowing your face into your pillow. These permanent creases crisscross over other lines and often occur on only one side of the face (usually the cheeks or chin). By sleeping on your back, you can prevent sleep lines.

4. "*Smoker's face*" is really two problems in one. First, the nicotine by-products from cigarettes can cause blood vessels to constrict, reducing vital oxygen flow (and other nutrients carried by the blood) to the skin. The result? Dull or sallow skin that lacks a healthy, rosy glow. Smokers also tend to develop deep "laugh lines" as well as fine wrinkles around the lips and eyes—possibly because of the puffing and squinting that occur when inhaling.

Smoking may also indirectly affect the amount of collagen that is being produced. Collagen is greatly responsible for keeping skin wrinkle-free. Collagen synthesis requires vitamin C, which is depleted by smoking. In fact, smokers need about 50 percent more vitamin C daily than non-smokers.

TURNING BACK THE CLOCK

Sunscreen is the first line of defense against aging skin, helping to prevent not only skin cancers, but wrinkles, "age" spots, dilated capillaries, uneven skin texture and tone, and sagging skin. What's more, some research indicates that skin that is protected from the sun for several years *may* actually begin to repair itself. (For more information on sunscreens, turn to pages 53-56.)

Alpha hydroxy acids are among the newest and most promising skin rejuvenators. Essentially compounds found in grapes, mangoes, apples, citrus fruits, and sour milk, among other things, these acids gently slough away dead cells on the skin's surface, then penetrate deep into the skin to effectively moisturize it. Early research indicates that alpha hydroxy acids *may* reduce fine lines and diminish age spots, and preliminary studies suggest they may also stimulate collagen formation so that aging or damaged skin can repair itself.

You'll find alpha hydroxy acids (particularly gly-

51

concolic acid in cosmetic ingredient labels) in newer, more advanced beauty treatments. Stronger formulations are available by prescription, and some dermatologists are using alpha hydroxy "peels" to reveal smoother, clearer, rosier skin in certain patients.

Liposomes are microscopic capsules containing moisturizing ingredients. These tiny "delivery systems" actually enhance the moisturization of the skin and soften and smooth it.

Retinol, retinoids, retinoic acid (Retin-A) are the antiacne formulas turned antiwrinkle treatments. Researchers feel that these topical vitamin A derivatives promote a faster turnover of cells and increased production of tiny blood vessels, giving skin a rosier glow, while "erasing" fine lines. Certain studies suggest that they also restore some of the skin's support (collagen and elastin) and resiliency to aging or sun-damaged skin, and some say they can lighten age spots.

These products start to visibly rid the skin of fine wrinkles within three to six months. They *can* sensitize the skin to sunlight, so wearing an SPF 15 sunscreen from morning until night is a must. Also, because there could be a tendency for the skin to dry, avoid using harsh soaps, exfoliating lotions, astringents, or cleansing grains.

As an antiwrinkle treatment, "vitamin A" products are a lifelong commitment: they work *only as long as you use them*. Stop and new wrinkles will appear.

VITAMIN "THERAPY" FOR YOUR SKIN

The success of Retin-A has promoted a flurry of research into the potential skin-beautifying benefits of other vitamin compounds.

"There's considerable controversy surrounding the effectiveness of vitamins incorporated into skin-care products such as sunscreens, moisturizers, eye gels, and lip balms," says Alex Znaiden, Director of Skin Care and Product Development for Avon. "The old thinking was that vitamins couldn't penetrate into the skin; new thinking says they *do*, and are available to be used by all layers of the skin, and this theory is supported by preliminary research findings at a number of universities," he adds.

Most promising are the "antioxidant" vitamins, A, C, and E, and beta carotene (a carotinoid, similar to vitamin A derivatives). According to Znaiden, the skin is constantly being attacked and damaged by "free radicals," highly charged energy molecules that form in— and on—the skin when it's exposed to ultraviolet rays, smog, and other forms of pollution. "Topically applied, the antioxidant vitamins are able to latch onto and deactivate these free radicals *before* they can harm your skin," Znaiden explains. He adds that free radicals can destroy the skin's collagen support system, resulting in sagging, wrinkling, and loss of elasticity.

Look for vitamins A, C, and E and beta carotene in sunscreens, moisturizers, eye creams, and lip preparations.

Bioflavonoids (sometimes referred to as "vitamin P") are also excellent antioxidants and show promise in protecting the skin from UV rays. "Bioflavonoids are highly effective antioxidant systems that protect *plants* from sun damage," explains Znaiden. "We think they work in a similar way to protect the skin from photoaging and are particularly useful in sunscreens, moisturizers, and eye gels."

Vitamin K is being incorporated into eye gels and creams. "Dark under-eye circles are often triggered by a leakage of blood from capillaries," notes Znaiden. "Sun exposure damages the capillaries and causes even more leakage. Vitamin K has been shown to strengthen blood vessels, and would be helpful in protecting them from sun damage."

SUN SENSE

Increasingly, Americans are becoming "sun smart," realizing that harmful ultraviolet (UV) rays are the skin's number one enemy, causing skin cancers, wrinkling, sagging, skin discoloration—and a host of other skin problems. The following is a skin-saving guide to protecting yourself from the sun.

UNDERSTANDING THE SPF SYSTEM

Sunscreen products are rated by an SPF (sun protection factor) number. SPFs tell how effectively a sunscreen blocks UVB rays (the so-called burning rays). To find out how long a particular product will protect you, multiply the SPF number on the label by the amount of time you can ordinarily spend in the sun (*without* sunscreen) before you begin to burn. If you usually start to turn pink in 20 minutes, an SPF 10 would allow you to spend 200 minutes (almost 3-1/2 hours) in the sun before burning begins. An SPF 15 screen would allow you to stay in the sun for 300 minutes.

SPF ratings refer *only* to protection from UVB rays—not to UVA rays (so-called tanning rays that researchers now know penetrate deeply into the skin to damage underlying structures and blood vessels, leaving skin wrinkled, leathery, and sagging). Sunscreens available today are formulated to protect against UVB radiation. According to the Skin Cancer Foundation, in New York City, most products rated SPF 15 or higher contain ingredients that provide *some* protection against UVA as well. To be on the safe side, the Foundation suggests you look for a broad-spectrum sunscreen containing one or more of these UVA-absorbers: oxybenzone; butyl methoxydibenzoylmethane; sulisobenzone; dioxybenzone; avobenzone; 2-Ethylhexyl 2-cyano-3; 3-diphenylacrylate; red petrolatum; titanium dioxide; zinc oxide.

FROM SUN UP TO SUN DOWN

The sun can damage your skin any time of the year. Although UVB rays aren't as strong during the winter, UVA rays are potent all year 'round. Protect yourself by wearing sunscreen that filters both UVB *and* UVA rays from morning until night (wear sunscreen under your makeup).

· UV rays are strongest between the hours of 10 AM and 3 PM. Schedule outdoor activities (tennis, jogging, swimming) in the early morning or late

54

afternoon, if possible—and do wear sunscreen on all exposed areas of the body.

·Everyday activities, like walking to and from work, spending an hour in the garden, taking a quick jog, call for a lightweight sunscreen or a moisturizer containing an SPF 15 sunscreen. (If your complexion is dark, you can get by with an SPF of 6 to 8.) *Serious* sunning—hours spent on a tennis court, at a pool, at the beach, or on the ski slopes—require sunscreens formulated for prolonged, direct exposure to the sun (opt for waterproof creams and lotions with high SPFs).

·For serious sunning, *slather* sunscreen on liberally. The average person should use about 1 ounce to coat all exposed areas of her body. Apply evenly to *dry* skin and rub in.

·Always apply sunscreen *at least 30 minutes prior* to sun exposure. Sunscreens must be absorbed into and react with the skin in order to protect it (they're *not* only a mechanical barrier that blocks UV rays by merely sitting on the skin's surface).

·Don't forget to coat your nose, ears, the back of your neck—and the backs of your hands. All are prime sites for skin cancers, and hands that are regularly exposed to the sun tend to get wrinkly and develop age spots as early as the late thirties!

· If you plan to swim or engage in a sport that will cause you to perspire, opt for a *waterproof* sunscreen. Regardless of the SPF rating, reapply the product every two or three hours—more often if you sweat profusely, or each time you towel dry your skin (sunscreens tend to rub off).

· Don't wait until you begin to turn pink to apply sunscreen. Damage to the skin begins long before a tell-tale burn starts to show.

· Choose the right sunscreen for your *skin type*. Dry and normal/combination complexions can generally tolerate oil or cream sunscreens. Oily and acne-prone skins call for non-comedogenic oil-free lotions or gels.

· In general, waterproof sunscreens in cream formulations tend to stay on the skin better than those in gel form. If you must wear a gel sunscreen (because you have acne, for example), reapply it frequently.

· As you age, your skin "thins"—and is more susceptible to sun-related damage. Choose higher-SPF products for added protection.

· Very "sun-sensitive" people may need extra-high-SPF formulations—15 or above.

· Some people are sensitive to certain ingredients in sunscreens, and may develop a rash, redness, itching, or tingling after applying a particular product. A small percent of the population is allergic to PABA (para-aminobenzoic acid) and its derivatives, including padimate-O and padimate-A. If you're "sunscreen-sensitive," experiment with several different formulations and look for ones labeled "hypoallergenic."

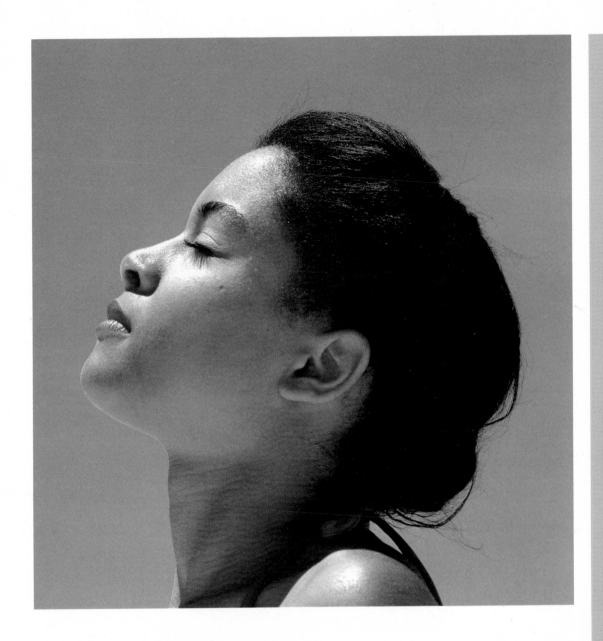

TO TAN—OR NOT

Is a tan *safe*? Actually, it's your skin's natural defense against sunburn (skin under UV attack forms extra melanin—or dark pigment—to protect itself). But a tan's level of protection is low, about the equivalent of an SPF 2 or 4 sunscreen. Tanned skin that's not protected by a broad-spectrum sunscreen *is* vulnerable to damage.

57

If you love the look of a tan, but want to spare your skin, opt for one of the new, improved self-tanning lotions (see "Self-Tan How-To's," page 103-04).

CROSS-COUNTRY BEAUTY

·Live in the *Midwest* or *Northeast*? Strong winter winds can dry out and redden any complexion. Shield the exposed areas of your face with a silk scarf instead of a wool muffler. Silk seals in warmth, won't irritate more sensitive skin as wool can.

·If you live in a super-dry or arid climate like the *Southwest*, drink six to eight glasses of water a day to replenish the moisture your skin naturally loses.

·Live in a sunny area like *Southern California*? Get into the habit of smoothing on an SPF 15 sunscreen *before* applying makeup—and do it year 'round!

·If you live in a region like the *Pacific Northwest*, which tends to be cloudy during much of the winter and spring, and even part of the summer, don't be fooled into thinking your skin's safe from the sun. UV rays can cut through a light cloud cover to damage unprotected skin. To be on the safe side, use moisturizer or foundation containing sunscreen. If you plan to spend more than 30 minutes outdoors, opt for an SPF 15 product.

BEAUTY WRAP-UP

1. Stop smoking. The nicotine by-products from cigarettes constrict blood vessels in the skin, reducing vital oxygen flow (and nutrients carried by the blood) to your skin's surface. The result? A dull, sallow complexion.

58

2. Use broad-spectrum sunscreens that block both UVB and UVA rays to prevent skin cancers as well as sun-related skin irregularities, like wrinkles, "age" spots, dilated capillaries.

3. Don't forget to use sunscreen on your nose, ears, and the backs of your hands—all prime sites for skin cancer.

CHAPTER

4

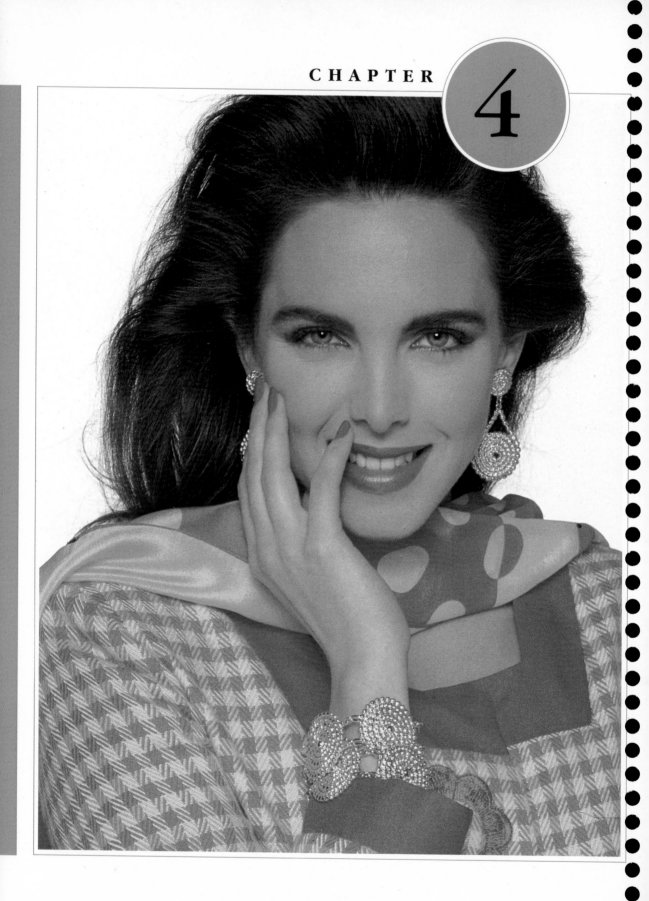

"I feel *naked* without makeup!"

Is this vanity talking? No, say psychologists, just a healthy sense of self-esteem. Whether they spend 2 minutes or 20 on their morning makeup routine, smart women realize that cosmetics can work a particular kind of magic, boosting self-confidence and influencing how others perceive them.

Makeups are *tools that transform*: they can minimize your beauty flaws, while maximizing your best features. Cosmetics can "wake up" a tired face, give warmth and glow to skin that's on the pale side, even out a splotchy complexion, conceal blemishes.

In the next three chapters, you'll see makeovers on women from all over the country. You will also discover hundreds of clever makeup tricks that will help you look—and feel—beautiful all day long.

TEST YOUR COLOR IQ

How many times has this happened to you? You buy a foundation or lipstick or blush thinking it will look wonderful—only to discover that it (a) washes you out, (b) makes you look like a clown, (c) looks fake or artificial.

Most of us have accumulated a drawer full of "wrong color" cosmetics at one time or another. But there are ways to take the guesswork out of buying makeup.

Complexions fall into one of two categories: *cool*, with a pinky-blue undertone, or *warm*, with a slightly yellow or golden underbase. If you're not sure which category you're in you'll want to determine whether you're a "cool" or a "warm," by gathering various items of clothing (solid-color scarves, blouses, sweaters, fabric remnants), and, if possible, two or more friends who can help you determine your complexion color type.

1. Divide fabric samples (wide enough to drape across shoulders) into two groups, each containing six (or more) of the following colors.

Faces of the Nineties

Group A: Look for blue-based colors—emerald green; sea green; deep red; soft raspberry; royal blue; cornflower blue; fuchsia; dusty rose; medium burgundy; purple.

Group B: Choose yellow-based colors—moss green; bright green; tomato red; medium orange; poppy; teal blue; turquoise; salmon; apricot or coral; lavender.

2. Cleanse your face of makeup and wrap your head in a white towel, covering your hair.

3. Working in natural daylight, drape yourself in fabrics in Group A, then Group B. Ask your friends to focus on your face, not on the fabric colors.

· When you're draped in the *right* colors, your complexion will look clearer, smoother, and your skin will have a healthy glow. Your eyes will take on a brighter appearance, and shadows and lines around your eyes and on cheeks will "fade." Your best colors will radiate a soft, flattering light under your jawline.

· The *wrong* colors will make you appear tired, sallow, or "washed out." Your eyes won't look as bright, and any lines or fine wrinkles and dark under-eye circles will be more noticeable. These colors will also cast a dark shadow under your jawline—and may even age you by five to ten years!

If you look best in Group A colors, your complexion tone is *cool*, with a pinky-blue undertone, and you should choose makeups in cool shades. If you look prettiest in Group B colors, your complexion is warm, with yellow undertones, and you should opt for makeups in *warm* tones.

FABULOUS FOUNDATION

Foundation is the most important cosmetic in a makeup artist's kit. The right foundation (keyed to your skin type and color) can even out skin tone and minimize splotchiness or patchy pigment. An oil-free

62

or water-based makeup will help keep oily skin from becoming shiny, while a moisturizing product will give dimension and dewy softness to dry skin that tends to look a little dull. Foundation provides the perfect "canvas" for eye makeup and blush, allowing them to smooth on like silk, stay color-true.

Here is a guide to choosing the best foundation for your particular skin type (to determine your skin type, see "Skin Typing," pages 25-26).

Dry Skin has a slightly "rough," lusterless look, plus a tendency toward slackness and tiny lines. Opt for a moisture-rich foundation in liquid or cream form, to plump up fine wrinkles, give skin glow (look for products containing light oils plus oil-free humectants like urea, which hold moisture to the skin all day long). For maximum hydration, always apply moisturizer *before* smoothing on foundation.

Oily Skin is hard on makeup. After just a few hours, oil will seep through, causing makeup to fade or change color. To sop up oil, use an alcohol- or witch-hazel-based astringent *before* applying foundation. Smooth an oil-free or gel moisturizer onto dry areas of face only (look for ones containing glycerin or urea). Choose oil-free, oil-blotting, water-based or matte foundations, or—for a very sheer base—a powder cream makeup (comes in a compact, smooths on with a sponge). Keep makeup color-true, prevent oil-breakthrough, by dusting face lightly with oil-absorbing translucent powder.

Midday shine? Pat away oil with special facial oil-blotting tissues, or pat a minimum of loose powder onto oily areas. Use a tissue or cotton ball to whisk away excess.

Normal/Combination Skin is generally oily in the T-zone, drier on the cheeks. Prep skin by whisking a cotton ball saturated in astringent across forehead, nose, and chin, then smooth a light lotion moisturizer over cheek areas only. Opt for a foundation formulated for "normal to oily" skin. (Note: Combination skin changes seasonally, becoming drier in the winter, oilier in the summer. See "Seasonal Switches," page 67, to find out how to "tailor" your makeup to fit the season.)

Blemished or Acne-Prone Skin needs special treatment. Since this complexion type is usually oily, prime skin with astringent, then smooth on a minimal amount of oil-free or water-based makeup. Look for products labeled "non-comedogenic" (which means they won't clog pores). Dust face lightly with oil-absorbing translucent powder. At midday, use oil-blotting tissues on oiliest areas of face, then lightly dust with translucent powder.

Sensitive Skin calls for makeups labeled "hypoallergenic," "allergy-tested," or "formulated for sensitive skin." Opt for sheer, fragrance-free products, and avoid makeups containing lanolin and those with alcohol high at the top of the ingredients list. Apply a minimal amount or use a damp makeup sponge for the sheerest coverage.

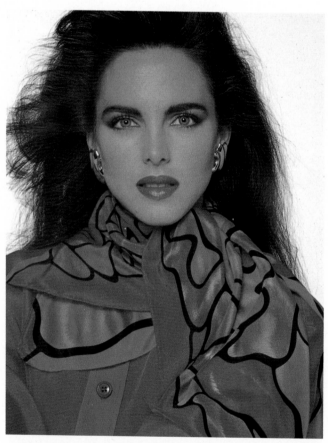

Many women can wear clothing from the warm and the cool groups. Always be sure to coordinate cosmetic shades to your wardrobe—whether it's warm.................

64

A PERFECT MATCH

Be sure to choose foundation that matches your skin tone exactly. Makeup that's too light will look chalky, mask-like. Too-dark foundation can pool in pores, make them appear larger, as well as accentuate fine lines and wrinkles. Foundation should complement your skin's undertone. Choose warm, "yellow-based" foundation if your complexion is warm, with a yellow or golden underbase. Opt for slightly "blue-based" makeup if your skin is cool, with a pinky-blue undertone.

· To find the right shade of makeup, apply a dab on your jaw. Don't test foundation on cheeks, nose,

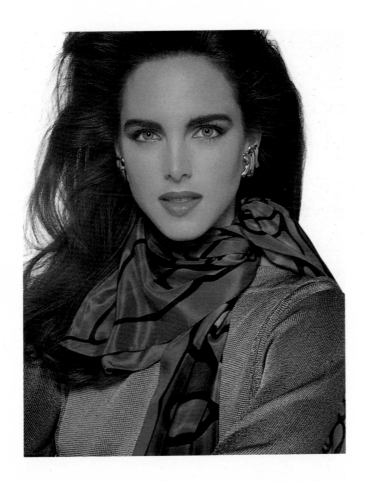

or cool.

or chin—these areas tend to be slightly ruddy, a little darker than the rest of your face. Testing makeup on your wrist won't give you a true match either, since the wrist area can be darker, more sallow than your facial skin.

· Fluorescent lighting (in drug and department stores) can distort the way makeup looks. Try to test foundation in natural light—by a window—if possible.

MAKEUP THAT MEETS SPECIAL NEEDS

If your skin's in good shape, but you need minimal coverage to even out skin tone and add warmth, opt for a *sheer* liquid or cream-powder foundation. But if you have large pores, blemishes, or fine lines that need concealing, choose a medium-coverage makeup in a creamier formulation. Oily skin plus large pores? Opt for a "pore-refining" product—essentially a "liquid powder" that creates a fine, matte finish.

Need to conceal a birthmark or scars (from acne or cosmetic surgery)? Choose an *opaque* concealing foundation (available in liquid and cream forms).

RED ALERT!

If you have a ruddy complexion—or are prone to rosacea, a common condition characterized by tiny dilated capillaries (usually visible on and around the nose, on the cheeks, and on the chin)—you'll need to color-correct your skin tone.

· Neutralize redness with a tinted moisturizer or makeup underbase in white, pale green, blue-white, or amber-yellow. Apply a minimal amount to reddish areas only and blend well before smoothing on foundation.

· Asian skin? Opt for a yellow-based or amber makeup primer.

66

·Black skin reddens first, then the red areas turn darker, giving your complexion a mottled look. Skip tinted primer; instead choose foundation *slightly* lighter than your skin tone and use a sponge to smooth on evenly.

A NATURAL LOOK

Foundation should look like your skin, not a "covering" for your complexion. For the most natural look:

1. Dot foundation onto forehead, nose, cheeks, and chin.
2. Using a *barely* damp makeup sponge, quickly spread and blend foundation downward and outward. Use sponge to blend foundation along and under jawline. (A dab on the eyelids can hold eyeshadow on longer.)
3. "Set" foundation and keep it from fading by dusting translucent powder over face and neck (use a big, fluffy brush or cotton puff). Whisk away excess with a cotton ball.
4. For a midday touch-up, pat a little pressed powder onto nose, cheeks, and chin.

SEASONAL SWITCHES

As the seasons change, so will your makeup needs. Use these smart, money-saving tricks to "transform" your foundation:

Dry skin: Needs extra moisture in the winter. Mix two fingertips of your regular hydrating foundation with a drop of moisturizer. Blend in the palm of your hand, then smooth over your face. In the summer, you'll need a lighter, sheerer base. Mix two fingertips of makeup with a tiny bit of water *or* a mini-pinch of translucent powder. Use a barely damp makeup sponge for smooth, sheer coverage.

Normal/combination skin: Gets parched in the winter. Add a drop of oil-free moisturizer to two fingertips of water-based or matte makeup to give your complexion a smoother, dewier look. In the summer,

Sallow Skin Warm-Up

Sallow complexions tend to look dull, sometimes unhealthy. Warm up sallow skin with a lavender underbase, then apply foundation.

67

curb your skin's natural tendency toward oiliness by mixing two fingertips water-based makeup with one fingertip of translucent powder.

Oily complexions are prone to a bit of flaking in the winter, so add a mini-drop of oil-free or gel moisturizer to your water-based or matte foundation. In the summer, create your own oil-absorbing foundation (that stays color-true!) by mixing two fingertips of oil-free makeup with one fingertip of oil-blotting loose powder.

WARMING BLACK SKIN

"Oil shows up more on black skin than on white or Asian complexions," says Tamara Friedman, President of the Institute de Beauté, in Detroit, Michigan. "Unless your skin is *very* dry, choose sheer oil-free or water-based foundation. Avoid creamier or thick formulations—they can look mask-like on black skin."

Also, check the ingredients label on foundation bottles (and on powder blush, eyeshadow, and sunscreen containers) to make certain the makeup *does not* contain titanium dioxide. "Black skin has a tendency to look ashy or grayish, and titanium dioxide will add to the ashiness," explains Friedman.

"Try to match your skin tone exactly when choosing foundation," she advises. "You may need to mix two colors to get an exact match." If your skin is very dark, it will probably have a warm reddish undertone. Look for foundation with a predominantly warm brown hue. Medium-toned skin may be on the sallow side. Opt for makeup with a hint of orange-red in the base to warm the skin. If your complexion is very light, it's likely to be a little sallow. Look for a delicate beige foundation with just a touch of red.

Powder is a must for black complexions, adding warmth, preventing an ashy look, minimizing shine. "Choose powder with care," advises Friedman. "Too-light shades or mauve or pink ones will emphasize ashiness, look artificial." Instead, select a powder that is very close to your foundation shade. Or you may need two powders that are close to your foundation shade—mix them in the palm of your hand to create a color that's a good match. Then, lightly dust over makeup and blend well.

Be sure to use oil-blotting tissues to pat away any oily shine.

MAKEUP FOR ASIAN BEAUTIES

"Asian skin can range from ivory to soft tan," notes Helen Lee, a professional model and owner of Helen Lee Skin Care, New York City. "But all Asian skin has a sallow or yellow underbase to varying degrees," she adds, "and many women make the mistake of trying to change their skin tone by using a pink-based foundation." The result? An artificial masky look. "The makeup will appear to be 'sitting' on the top of your skin, it'll look like a layer of pink powder," Lee observes.

"For the most natural look, use a sheer liquid base and match your skin tone exactly. A foundation with a yellow underbase will actually warm and enhance Asian skin.

"To 'rosy up' your complexion, rely on pink- or rose-toned blushes in either cool or warm shades," she adds. (See "Enhancing Asian Cheeks and Lips," page 94.)

POWDER POWER

Powder is a makeup artist's secret weapon. They'll use it to even skin tone, "set" foundation, to soften and change makeup.

·Choose powder keyed to your skin type. If your skin is *dry*, opt for a moisturizing pressed or loose powder. *Oily* skin? Look for an oil-absorbing loose powder. *Normal/combination* complexion? Any loose or pressed powder will work for you.

·"Tinted" powders can color-correct skin-tone problems. Use a yellow-based or golden powder to give glow to pale skin that's got a warm or yellowish undertone. Opt for an opal or blush-pink powder to warm fair skin that's on the cool side (with a pinky-blue undertone). Choose a sheer mauve-toned powder to take the yellow out of sallow skin.

· To change your lipstick from shiny to matte in an instant, apply lip color, then dust loose translucent powder over lips.

· To keep under-eye liner from smudging, dip a cotton swab into loose powder, then gently brush over line. Use clean end to dust away excess.

· For fade-proof cheek color, smooth foundation over skin, then dust with translucent powder. Apply blush, *then* lightly dust powder *over* blusher.

· Dust loose powder over eyeshadow after applying. It'll keep shadow from fading or smudging; helps turn a frosted shadow to a matte.

BEAUTY WRAP-UP

1. Match foundation to skin tone. Test makeup in *natural* light on your jaw to find the color closest to your skin shade.

2. If your skin has a pinky-blue undertone, choose "cool" colors. Skin that has a yellow or golden undertone calls for "warm" makeup shades.

3. Choose foundation that's right for your skin *type*, but remember that skin type can change with the seasons—and you'll need to change your makeup accordingly.

4. Use powder to "finish" and perfect your look. But don't overdo. A light dusting will leave your skin fresh, shine-free.

5. If you have black skin, match powder to your foundation shade for a warm, natural look. Avoid too-light or pink or mauve-based powders, which can look artificial on darker skin.

6. Avoid using pink-based foundation on Asian skin; it will look like pink powder, sitting on top of the skin. Instead, choose a yellow-based makeup to give skin natural-looking warmth.

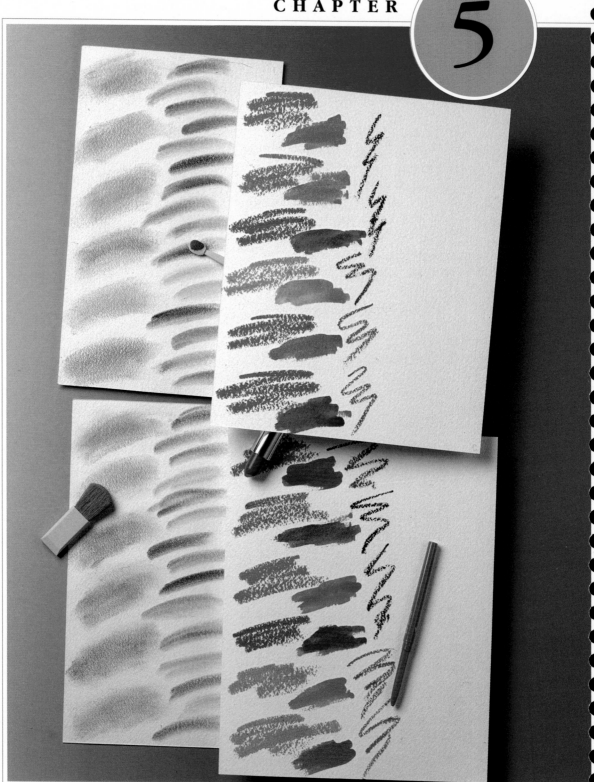

CHAPTER 5

With a lot of know-how—and a little practice—you can learn to apply makeup like the pros.

ZERO IN ON YOUR BEST FEATURE

Most makeup artists agree that you should focus on—or draw attention to—your best feature and away from any flaws. If your lips are full and luscious, play them up with brighter lip colors, while applying more neutral shades to cheeks and eyes. If you're blessed with a wide-eyed look, choose makeup colors that will enhance your eyes, opting for more subtle hues for lips and cheeks. High cheekbones? Use blush to contour, emphasize your cheeks, while selecting softer, muted colors for lips and eyes.

Whatever you do, don't highlight lips, cheeks, *and* eyes. You can end up looking like a clown, and others won't focus on any one part of your face.

FOCUS ON EYES

Check out these tips for foolproof eye makeup:

1. To keep eyeshadow from fading, "prime" lids with a lid fixative or a hint of foundation.

2. To add dimension to eyes, use eyeliner pencil, drawing a fine line along upper lashes (stay close to lash base), from about 1/4 inch from the inside corner to the outside corner of eye. Use your little finger or a small sponge-tip applicator to smudge slightly. If you opt for a line beneath lower lashes, be sure to stay *under* lashes—don't line the insides of eye rims; you'll risk infection (as well as "closing in" the eye). Starting at center of eye, just below middle of pupil, draw a very fine line to outer corner and smudge slightly. To "set" lower line, dip a sponge-tip applicator into loose powder and dust over line, or apply a medium to deep-tone eyeshadow (just a hint!) using a sponge-tip applicator edge.

Makeup Lessons

73

3. Stroke medium- to darker-tone eyeshadow onto outer edge of lid and into crease area (for a "three-dimensional" look, use a darker shadow in crease of the eye).

4. Smooth lighter shadow over lids and onto browbones.

5. Apply two coats of mascara for thickest, longest lashes. Holding wand in a vertical position, use tip to color ends of lashes, sweeping brush back and forth like a windshield wiper. Turn wand to horizontal position and sweep upward through lashes, wiggling the brush back and forth to coat "sides" of each lash. To remove excess mascara, gently blot with tissue. Or, use a lash comb to separate lashes, remove any mascara clumps.

6. Apply one coat of mascara to bottom lashes. (Be sure to use a waterproof, smudge proof formula to prevent racoon eyes!)

MORE EYE-OPENING TIPS

· For long-lasting shadow that doesn't fade or accumulate in the crease of the eye, opt for a pressed-powder shadow. Lightly dust lids with translucent powder after stroking on shadow. If you prefer a cream shadow, top with powder shadow or translucent powder.

· Dust lashes with a bit of translucent powder before applying mascara to boost its staying power (don't use powder on lashes if you wear contact lenses).

· Use a cotton swab or cosmetic sponge with a dot of foundation to wipe away mascara, shadow, or liner smudges beneath eyes.

· If shadow begins to fade halfway through the day, gently press tissue against lids to blot up oil and moisture. Then, reapply shadow.

· If liner pencil's too hard and doesn't glide on easily (a common complaint during colder months),

74

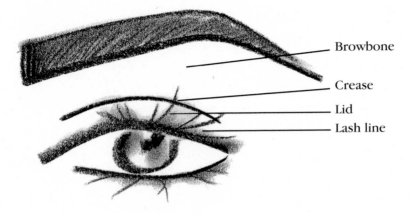

Browbone

Crease

Lid

Lash line

hold tip between your fingers for a few seconds. Pencil too soft? Refrigerate overnight for greater precision when applying. (Refrigeration helps "prime" pencils for sharpening, too.)

·Skimpy lashes? Gently curl lashes and apply two coats of lash-thickening mascara, allowing first coat to dry before applying second.

BEAUTIFUL-BROW KNOW-HOW

The length of your brows should be in proportion to the rest of your features, and brows should start just above the inner corner of your eye and extend slightly past the outer corner.

If your brows extend into the area between your eyes, pluck stray hairs. Moisten a cotton ball with mild astringent and gently wipe brow area to help prevent infection. Using slant-edged tweezers, pluck one hair at a time in *direction of hair growth*. To minimize irritation, smooth a little moisturizer over brows after plucking. (You may want to have a professional give you an initial brow shaping—by tweezing or waxing. You'll have an easier time following the line, thereafter.)

Be conservative when removing hair from the brow area. Brows that have been waxed, tweezed, or shaved too frequently won't always grow back.

Fill in sparse brows by adding a little color to area

75

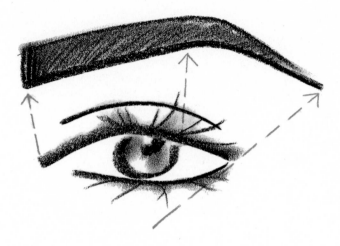

nearest nose, then comb or brush upper edge of brow hairs for "lift." (This technique will also "open up" your eyes.) Brow pencils and brush-on brow powders are good bets.

Bushy brows? Use "clear" mascara to comb brows upward, hold them in place. Or, mist a brow brush or old toothbrush with hairspray (or rub a tiny dab of setting gel over bristles) and use to comb brows up and outward.

LENS ALERT

Wear contact lenses? Avoid *very* powdery shadows, or those that contain metallic or glittery ingredients, which can flake into eyes, causing irritation. Opt for stick, pencil, or creamy powder shadows.

Steer clear of lash-lengthening or thickening mascaras that contain "fibers" designed to extend lashes. The fibers can get trapped between your lens and your eye, triggering irritation and possible damage to the cornea. Instead, look for mascaras *formulated for contact-lens wearers* (these products are generally smudgeproof, waterproof, and flakeproof).

Always insert contact lenses *before* applying eye makeup; otherwise, you risk smudging your makeup, as well as getting mascara flakes into eyes.

Use a non-oily eye makeup remover or baby shampoo to remove eye makeup thoroughly. Avoid

76

oily products—they can leave a greasy film around the eye, which will coat lenses when you re-insert them. (Note: Remove lenses *before* taking off eye makeup.)

Don't use cotton balls or cotton swabs near eyes. The cotton fibers can stick to your lenses; opt for sponge applicators instead.

PROBLEM SOLVERS

To keep *deep-set eyes* from disappearing, arch brows slightly. Contour browbone with a subtle, medium to dark shadow. Smooth a lighter shadow (iridescent for evening) onto lid and into crease. Avoid dark shadows on lids, steer clear of dark or thick eye liner.

To minimize *too-prominent eyes*, apply dark matte shadow on lid, extending color into crease. Use highlighter just under brow. Using dark liner, draw a thick line on upper lid (don't extend past outer corner). Smudge slightly. Draw a thin line under lower lashes, from center to outer corner. Eyebrows should have a well-defined arch, peaking just beyond center of eye.

Make *small eyes* look bigger by applying a subtle dusting of blush from hairline to just above outer corner of brow. Use a fine-tipped pencil to line eyelid from center to outer corner and smudge slightly. Apply light-toned or lightly frosted shadow onto lid, stopping at crease (use matte for day, iridescent shades for evening). Draw a fine line beneath lower lashes at outer corner only. Stroke one coat of mascara onto lashes, then apply a second coat to outer half of lashes only. Keep brows neat and on the thin side so they don't "overpower" your eyes.

Widen *close-set eyes* by smoothing a light cream concealer or powder highlighter on area between nose and eye, extending it from bottom of eye up to inner brow. Apply shadow to lid, starting at center of eye and blending it up and out toward the end of the brow. Pluck brows from underneath to create more space between brows and eyes; brows should start just beyond inner corners of eyes, peak slightly above centers of pupils, and end just past the outer corners of eyes.

Minimize *bulging eyes* by using a soft thick pencil

in brown or gray, above upper lashes and beneath lower ones. Use brown or gray shadow on lids, from lashline to crease. Holding mascara wand in a vertical position, apply color to upper halves or tips of lashes.

Bring *wide-set eyes* closer together by applying a dark-toned shadow between nose and eye, blending very well. Beginning at inner corner of the eye, stroke eyeliner close to lashes, stopping just before you reach the outer corner. Brows should start a little closer to the nose, in order to decrease space between eyes.

To detract from *hidden lids* (where very little lid shows), stroke a light, clear shadow over lid. Smudge a smoky-toned shadow into crease, slanting it slightly up and out, just beyond the outer corner of the eye. Apply a lighter shadow (ivory, pink, pale peach) over the inner corners of the eye, just under the brow. Apply two coats of mascara. Pluck brows from underneath and use a brow pencil to extend them just a bit at the outer corners. (Heavy brows can weigh down this eye shape!)

To camouflage *crepy eyelids*, stick with muted matte shadows. Avoid frosted or iridescent ones—they'll magnify the fine lines.

GORGEOUS BLACK EYES

"Sometimes, a black woman's eyes will appear tired because the whites take on a yellowish hue," says Detroit makeup and skin-care pro Tamara Friedman. "Avoid using brown liner pencils, which can intensify the yellow tinge. Instead, choose 'eye-brightening' colors like gray, black, and midnight blue," she advises, adding that "Almond-shaped eyes look beautiful on black women. You can create the illusion of 'almond eyes' by using a jade green or violet pencil to highlight the outer corners of eyes (draw a little triangle)."

Don't use black pencil to fill in or shape brows, says Friedman. The black can take on a gray appearance. Instead, opt for brow pencil in brown-black for a natural look.

Depending on the depth of your skin tone, you can experiment with many shadow hues. "Earth tones work well on medium- to light-black skin, while brights and jewel tones (medium burgundy, berry, sapphire, dark coral) are striking—but not garish—on darker complexions. The dark skin tone 'mutes' brighter colors, giving them a subtler appearance," explains Friedman.

ASIAN EYE APPEAL

"Asians have beautiful eyes," says makeup expert Helen Lee. "Don't try to change your eyes by drawing an artificial crease onto the lid. Instead, enhance their natural beauty with these tricks":

· Opt for a natural look, using shadows in the brown family (neutral colors like khaki look especially pretty on Asian eyes).

· Define your lids by lining the top lid with dark brown or charcoal liner. Don't use black liner under lower lashes—your eyes are so dark they'll make a black line look hard, artificial. Instead, use a soft brown pencil to draw a subtle line beneath lower lashes.

· If your eyes are *almond-shaped*, create a graduated line on the lid, very narrow at the inner corner and widening gradually over the pupil and becoming fairly thick at the outer corner. Smudge to soften.

· Very *narrow* eyes? Use black or deep purple liner along upper lashes, then dust the lid area with a shadow three to four shades darker than your skin color (good choices— taupe, deep coral). Apply mascara.

· If your eyelids appear puffy because there's no visible crease or fold in the lid, create the illusion of a *slight* crease by using dark brown shadow on the lower part of the lid, but gradually softening (or lightening) it as you continue sweeping color up to brow. (Color should be darkest near lashes, palest near brows.) Avoid shiny or "frosted" shadows— they'll emphasize puffiness.

COLOR MAGIC

Here's what shadow can do for your eyes!

Eye Color	Shadow Color	Effect
Blue	Brown Pink Plum Gray	Intensifies blue, makes eyes bright, clear.
Green/Hazel	Yellow (mustard) Orchid Sand Topaz	Brings out gold in hazel eyes, brightens green.
Brown	Mauve Olive Tan Sapphire	Enriches depth and warmth of brown eyes through contrast.
Black	Plum Tan (or khaki) Blue Pink	Draws attention to eye and brightens eye area.

RX FOR COMMON EYE PROBLEMS

Problem: **Your lashes are falling out.**

Possible Causes:
· Using old, dried-out mascara.
· Not completely—or gently—removing all eye make-up at bedtime.
· Using a dirty or damaged eyelash curler on a daily basis.

Solutions:
· Replace mascara every two to three months.
· Use eye-makeup remover nightly (*especially* if you use waterproof mascara).
· Opt for mascara with a special rounded wand that *curls* lashes, as well as colors them. Don't rely on metal curlers, which can break lashes—even pull them out.

Problem: **Your mascara is "clumpy."**

Causes:	· Applying too much mascara in first application.
	· Not allowing mascara to dry between applications.
Solutions:	· Apply one thin coat of mascara. Allow to dry. Apply a second coat.
	· Use an eyelash comb to separate lashes, remove clumps.
Problem:	**Mascara smudges under eyes.**
Causes:	· Using too much moisturizer, moisturizing foundation, or creamy concealer under eyes.
	· Glasses frames that rest on cheeks.
Solutions:	· Blot under-eye area with tissue to remove excess oil. Dust on a little translucent powder.
	· Make sure glasses frames are supported by the bridge of your nose—*not* your cheeks. If frames rest on cheeks, moisture, oil, and perspiration can accumulate under lenses, cause makeup smudging.
Problem:	**Your mascara flakes off.**
Cause:	· The product is old and dry.
Solution:	· Replace mascara every two to three months—sooner if it appears to be drying out.
Problem:	**Your eyeshadow "creases" on your lids.**
Causes:	· Oily lids.
	· Using pencil or cream shadow alone.
Solutions:	· Apply powder eyeshadow in a similar shade *over* pencil or cream formulation to "set."
Problem:	**Your shadow fades by midday.**
Cause:	· Improper application.
Solutions:	· Dust lids with loose powder *after* applying shadow.
	· Use a sponge-tip applicator, rather than a brush, for more intense color.
	· Smooth a shadow "base" or foundation over lids, then top with powder shadow.
Problem:	**You have dark circles under your eyes.**
Causes:	· Heredity.

81

· Lack of sleep.
· Using wrong makeup shades.
· Rubbing eyes.

Solutions:
· *Before* applying makeup, soothe eyes by placing any of the following on them for 3 to 5 minutes: cool potato slices, cool cucumber slices, cooled damp chamomile tea bags, big cotton puffs soaked in cool milk.
· Apply foundation. Then, use fingertip to pat concealer, half a shade lighter than your normal skin color, onto dark areas only. Choose concealer with a *yellow underbase* to neutralize the purple-red hue in the dark circles. Blend carefully.
· Dust, don't press, a little loose powder over concealer to "set." Even and blend by running your little-finger tip gently around rim of eyesocket.
· Don't use mauve, pink, or purple shadows—they'll intensify dark circles.
· Never rub your eyes—and *do* get a good night's sleep!

Problem:
You wake up with puffy eyes (especially in under-eye area).

Causes:
· Allergies, like hay fever.
· Fluid retention.

Solutions:
· Check with your doctor to see if an allergy medication (antihistamine) is in order.
· Restrict intake of very salty foods—or packaged foods containing high amounts of sodium, which can promote fluid retention.
· Realign your bed so your head is higher than your feet, or sleep with two pillows. By elevating your head, you can minimize the accumulation of fluid in the eye area.
· Use cool compresses (see above in "dark under-eye circles" solutions) to reduce puffiness.
· Use eyeliner along top lashes, but *not* under lower ones. Smooth foundation below eyes, then, using pressed powder in a shade that matches skin tone, pat onto under-eye area, down onto cheeks. This method will "erase" the puffs.
· Puffy lids? Use a light-gray pencil along upper lashes. Opt for subdued matte shadow—frosted shadows will emphasize puffiness.

82

Problem: **Your eyes are red-rimmed.**

Causes:
· An allergy or cold.
· You've been crying.

Solutions:
· Take the red out with cool compresses (see list in "dark under-eye circles" section).
· Neutralize redness by using a baby blue or cornflower blue pencil to draw a fine line close to upper lashes, beneath lower ones. Slightly smudge both lines. Opt for shadows that counteract redness: jade green, brown, khaki. Avoid red-based shadows like fuchsia, burgundy, wine, plum or pink—they'll play up the red hue.

EYE ART FOR GLASSES WEARERS

· Nearsighted? Your eyes will look smaller—may disappear—behind lenses. Wear more makeup to play up and define eyes. Opt for pale, but vibrant, shades of shadow on lids and use liner on lids and beneath lower lashes. Two coats of mascara are a must!

· Farsighted? Your eyes will look larger through lenses. Be discreet with makeup; choose subtle matte shadow; and line top lashes only—if at all. Go easy on mascara—one coat may be enough.

· Use concealer under eyes; glasses magnify dark circles and lines.

· Opt for smudgeproof mascara—it won't "grease up" lenses.

GETTING FRAMED

Choose glasses that flatter but *don't match* your face shape, and keep in mind your hairstyle when selecting the frames.

· *Round face:* Opt for thick, angular frames with a

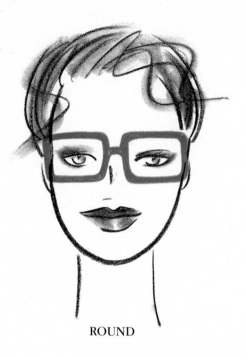

ROUND

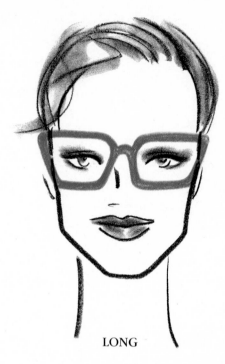

LONG

slight upward tilt on top—they'll "lengthen" your face. Avoid rimless or transparent styles that "get lost" on your face.

·*Long face:* Choose frames that are wider than your cheekbone area to create an illusion of width.

·*Square face:* Go for upswept "cat's-eyes" frames or oval or round shapes. Both will soften the contours of your face.

·*Heart-shaped face:* Opt for geometrics, ovals, rectangular, or square-shaped frames. Avoid "aviator" shapes.

·*Small face:* Don't overwhelm your features with over-sized or heavy frames. Choose thin metal-rimmed styles that allow your beauty to show through.

·*Long nose:* "Shorten" with frames that have a high side-bar, drawing attention upward toward temples—and away from your nose.

84

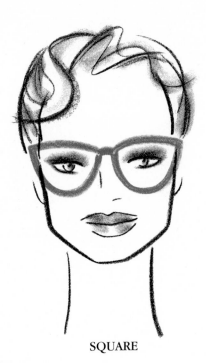

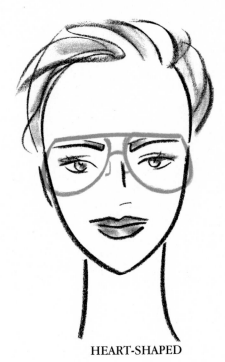

SQUARE   HEART-SHAPED

·*Short hair:* Try subtle, light designs or round frames that don't overwhelm your face.

·*Long, full hair:* Rimless or feminine frame shapes will flatter and complement the soft contours of your hair shape.

·*Hairstyles with bangs:* Be sure bangs stay clear of the rims. Avoid dark, thick frames that can create shadows around the eyes and face.

·*Severe styles or hair pulled off the face:* Enjoy bolder frames with unique shapes to soften the hairstyle.

·*Young, trendy haircuts:* Go for dramatic shapes and colors to emphasize your look.

COLOR KEY

The frames of your glasses should complement your skin tone and hair color.

·*Fair or rosy complexion, blonde or light brown hair:* Try frames in pink, blue, plum, lavender, silver, gray, or pewter.

·*Dark, golden or olive skin, brown or black hair:* Look for frames in dark coral, brown, medium to dark tortoise shell, gold or bronze.

·*Fair skin, red hair:* Opt for frames in light or dark tortoise shell, dark pastels, even black.

·*Fair skin, gray hair:* Choose frames in lavender, peach, pink, blue-violet, gold.

·*Olive skin, gray hair:* Opt for frames in burgundy, garnet, silver, or pewter.

BLUSHING BEAUTY

Properly applied, blush will give your face warmth, natural glow, and "heighten" your cheekbones. Check out your cheek color the next time you exercise—their natural rosy shade is the one you want to match when you look for blusher.

Enhancing your complexion with blush (or "rouge," as it was once called) can be achieved with either powder or cream formulations. Cream blushes are best for older women or those with very dry skin. Powder forms are a must for women who have oily complexions. (Powder blush tends to go on easier and last longer than creams.)

WAYS TO BLUSH

1. Smile to locate the "apples" of your cheeks; then apply blush onto apples, blending "edges" with a cotton puff or sponge.

2. Apply blush high on cheeks. Don't make the mistake of applying color *under* the cheeks, thinking it will give the illusion of "high cheekbones." This will only make your face look fuller.

3. Smooth blush up and out, starting just under

Real Beauty . . . Real Women

the center of the eye, then sweeping color lightly up into hairline for a natural look.

4. Frame your face with color by lightly applying blush along the jaw. Blend well to avoid an obvious look.

5. Extend a bit of color over the bridge of nose (especially pretty when using tawny or coral blushes for a "sun-kissed" look); avoid doing this if your skin is ruddy, however.

MORE CHIC CHEEK TIPS

·Avoid uneven blush, splotchy-looking or over-colored cheeks. Apply blush in natural daylight, using a big, fluffy brush. Tap brush on the back of your hand to remove excess color before stroking blush onto cheeks.

·For true-to-life cheek color, "layer" two shades of blush. First fluff on a soft peach shade, then top with a soft pink for a naturally tawny-rosy look.

·Pale, translucent skin? Avoid true-pink colors, which can look pasty, artificial. Instead, choose colors with a slightly blue undertone—pale tones of plum, rose, soft berry—if your skin's on the cool side. Warm-toned skin? Opt for yellow-based blush in dusty peach, soft rose or apricot.

·Very ruddy cheeks or dilated capillaries? Use a green, white, or yellow base under foundation, and/or opt for yellow-based blush colors like tawny peach, rose-brown, or, for dark skins, deep cinnamon.

·Olive-skinned beauties should avoid too pale or too pink blush, which can appear artificial. Instead, choose shades of dark peachy-coral, deep tawny-rose, medium burgundy, plum.

·Change your blush with the seasons. Opt for dustier or softer colors during the fall and winter, lighter, brighter shades for spring and summer.

87

· For a pulled-together look, *always* choose blush and lipstick in the same color family.

· Keep blush color-true by applying foundation, then lightly dusting cheeks with translucent powder. Dust on blush, then fluff on a little more powder, and blend well.

· If your skin's oily, avoid cream or frosted powder blushes—they'll add shine to skin (and creams will quickly fade). Opt for powder cheek color for a matte look.

· Dry cheeks? *Some* powder blushes can look "cakey," as if they're sitting on top of your skin. Opt for moisture-rich powder blush, or creamy moisturizing stick blush for dewy-looking color. Another good bet: cream blush, which gives cheeks a soft, radiant look.

· Wrinkly cheeks? Avoid frosted blushes—they'll emphasize the lines.

· For blush that goes on super-smoothly (and stays put), dip brush into loose powder, pat on back of hand to remove excess, then stroke across blush color-pad. Sleek color onto cheeks.

When applying blush, remember that light or frosted shades will make an area more prominent. Dark tones can cause an area to recede. For the illusion of high cheekbones, use lighter (or iridescent) blush along top of cheekbone, a medium- or darker-toned shade directly on cheekbone, blending together with lighter shade.

LIP LINES

What's the most frequently used item in a woman's makeup kit? Lipstick! Chances are, you apply—or freshen—your lip color two, three, four times a day. But many women don't apply lipstick correctly—or use it to make the most of their looks. Here, a guide to luscious lips.

1. Apply foundation or lip toner onto lips.
2. Outline shape of mouth with pencil.
3. Fill in with coordinating color (be sure to cover liner).
4. Blot center of lips lightly and reapply color.

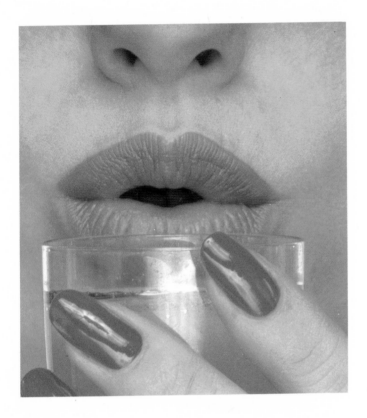

If your lips are less than perfect, you can redefine or reshape your mouth with these clever tricks:

Too-full lips: Smooth a tiny amount of foundation over mouth. Line just inside natural lip line to outer corners. Opt for medium or dark matte lipstick, applying to lips and into penciled area. Avoid: glosses, frosteds, or bright colors.

Thin lips: Using lip liner in a shade that's close to your lipstick color, *or* in "nude," draw a fine line along the outer edges of your natural lip line. Use light- to medium-bright lipstick and dot gloss onto bottom lip. It'll reflect light onto upper lip, and your mouth will look fuller. Opt for iridescent lip color for evening.

Thin upper lip: Draw a fine line just outside natural line of upper lip. Use a slightly lighter or brighter lip color on upper lip, a darker one on lower lip. Press lips together to blend colors.

Too-full upper lip: Use lip liner along inside of up-

Brush Strokes

Lip brushes offer precision application (that's why makeup artists rely on them!). Choose a brush with short, firm bristles. To pick up color, use long gentle strokes along the sides of your lipstick (that way, the lipstick will retain its shape). Brush color evenly onto lips. (If you prefer to apply lip color directly from the tube, be sure not to swivel lipstick up more than 1/2 inch—or you risk breaking it off.)

per lip. Use a darker shade of lipstick on upper lip, a slightly paler one on lower lip. Press lips together to blend color.

Droopy lips: Smooth foundation over corners of mouth. Use lip pencil to lightly and subtly extend corners of lip upward. Apply lipstick.

Too-wide lips: Smooth foundation over outer corners of mouth. Line lips, keeping just inside natural line. Don't extend liner to outer corners. Apply your regular lipstick, then, using lipstick in the same color family—but brighter than your regular shade—smooth onto center of mouth. Blot with tissue to blend the two colors.

Lopsided lips: Pat foundation over lip edge, then use a pencil to draw a fine line slightly outside scanty lip line, so it matches the other half.

LIP TRICKS

· Make lips look fuller by smoothing gloss over a light—or bright—lipstick.

· Line lips with pencil that matches your lipstick or is a *hint* darker. (Or, opt for a nude pencil liner.) The line shouldn't be obvious.

· Use a touch of iridescent highlighter in the groove above upper lip to accentuate a pretty "cupid's bow."

· For a shiny look, rub a little mineral oil or a dab of petroleum jelly over lips before applying color.

· Need a super-natural, semi-matte look that really stays put? Smooth a *little* petroleum jelly or gloss over lips. Using a lip pencil in an earthy tone (rosy-brown, cinnamon, dusty peach, terra cotta), outline lips, then use pencil to color in the rest of lip area. Dab a dot of gloss onto center of lower lip and press lips together.

· Prevent lipstick from "feathering" into fine lines around your mouth by smoothing a lip fixative or

90

lip toner over mouth and slightly outward around lip line. Allow to "soak in" for one minute. Then, outline lips in a neutral shade (or use pencil that matches lipstick). Apply one coat of lipstick, gently pat with tissue, then dust lips with a minimum of translucent powder.

· Teeth looking a little yellow? To make teeth look whiter, choose cooler lip colors in clear blue-reds, roses, burgundy. Avoid yellow-based colors like orange, browns, cinnamon, peach, apricot.

· Lipstick "sticks"—doesn't glide on when you've been outdoors and your mouth is cold? Before touching up lip color, cup your hand over mouth for a few seconds and blow in and out to warm lips. Lipstick will go on smoothly.

· If your lipcolor turns "blue" on lips, opt for colors with a "yellow" base: corals, peach tones, browns, cinnamon.

· Don't cake on more lipstick at midday—you'll end up with too much color in some areas, not enough in others. Instead, tissue lips to wipe away color. Smooth on a *hint* of lip fixative and blot lips with tissue. Reapply lip color.

· Don't pucker up—or stretch your lips into a wide smile—when lining lips. Instead, relax mouth, then draw a fine line around lip edges.

LIP SAVERS (FOR CHAPPED OR SORE LIPS)

Smooth a moisturizing lip balm over lips before applying color. Lip balms will smooth the rough surface on chapped lips, allow color to go on evenly. To keep lipstick from looking "cakey," rub a little color onto your fingertip, then pat over lips. Opt for moisture-rich lipsticks; matte colors will cake, look patchy on chapped, dry lips.

Cold sore or fever blister? Avoid applying lip color directly on the sore area—you risk further infection, and you can contaminate your lipstick. To dry up cold sores quickly, ask your pharmacist to recommend a protective, drying agent that forms a "seal" over the sore. To color lips, rub lipstick onto fingertip, then smooth on unaffected areas of mouth. Avoid too-bright, too-dark, or frosted colors—they'll call attention to your mouth. To detract from a cold sore, opt for super-natural shades that give lips a minimum of color: soft peach, rosy-brown, dusty apricot.

The sun's rays can burn delicate lip tissue—and a burn can trigger fever blisters. To prevent both, coat lips with a lip balm or lip color containing an SPF 15 sunscreen whenever you plan to spend more than 30 minutes outdoors.

MAKEUP FOR YOUR FACE SHAPE

Your face shape determines which features you should accent, those you should minimize. Below, tips for five common face shapes:

Oval: Forehead is wider than the chin, cheekbones are dominant. Nothing should detract from the

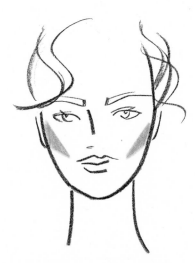

Blush or contouring applied in an upward and outward diagonal can make a full face appear narrower.

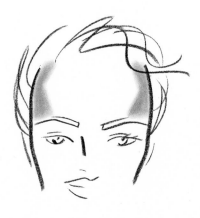

Narrow a wide forehead and temple area with a foundation or shading powder a little darker than your skin tone.

beautiful line of your face, so keep makeup subtle. Eyebrows should be neat and arched.

Round: Forehead is rounded, as are chin and jaw lines. Cheeks are full. To slim "plump" cheeks, arch eyebrows *slightly* and use makeup to play up eyes. Apply shadow, making sure it doesn't extend beyond outer corners of eyes. Concentrate mascara toward center of eyes. Blush must be applied carefully in a triangle high on cheeks, then blended outward, ending one inch or so before hairline. Follow natural lip line; do not extend.

Triangle/heart: Forehead is broad, cheeks are full. The face narrows to a pointed chin. To balance the face, creating wideness at the bottom, arch brows slightly and apply highlighter high on cheeks in a triangular shape. Just below highlighter, use blush to create another triangle. Blend edges well. A "dot" of blush on the chin will soften "pointy" effect. Opt for pale or neutral lip colors. Keep lip line, lips, full.

Square: The forehead is squared and the same width as cheekbones and jaw. To slightly soften the geometric line of your face, opt for subtle makeup. Eyebrows shouldn't have a harsh line, but can be slightly arched. Emphasize eyes with shadow, liner,

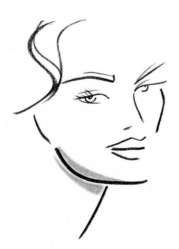

Shading just below the jawline can diminish a slack jawline or double chin.

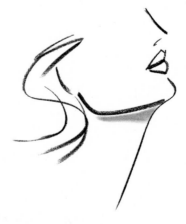

Slenderize the upper neck and jowl area by applying shading upwards along the jawline.

93

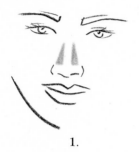

1.

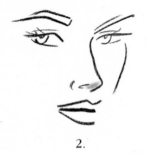

2.

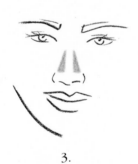

3.

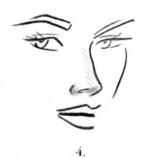

4.

and mascara. Apply blush on cheekbones, sweeping color outward, then down. Smooth blush along jawline to soften edges.

Rectangle/oblong: Similar to the square face, but slightly elongated. The forehead is high, cheeks are long and hollow. The jaw is slightly squared. To shorten and soften the line of your face, arch brows slightly and apply blush high on cheekbones and outward. The lip lines should be wide and full, the lips tinted with a pale or subtle color. A dash of tawny or rosy-brown blush on the chin will help shorten your face.

MORE FACE SHAPERS

1. If your nose is too broad at the bridge or base, narrow it by drawing triangles of foundation (or matte powder) two or three shades deeper than your usual color, on either side of the wide area (tip of triangle should be at top). Blend into rest of makeup.

2. To shorten a long nose, dot a tiny amount of darker foundation or powder on the end of nose and blend well.

3. To straighten a crooked nose, apply a darker-toned foundation or powder along the crooked side, a lighter one on the other side. Blend well.

4. To reshape a flat nose with a broad base, use foundation slightly lighter than your skin tone to smooth a line right down the center of the nose. Apply darker foundation on nostrils. Blend well.

ENHANCING ASIAN CHEEKS AND LIPS

"Asian women are fortunate because most can wear either cool *or* warm lip and cheek colors," says makeup pro Helen Lee, noting that cool colors create a soft, feminine look, while warm tones offer a natural, subtle beauty.

94

"If your skin is *very* sallow, try cool blush and lip colors from blue-pinks to blue-burgundies, depending on how light or dark your skin is," she suggests. "The yellow undertone in your complexion will neutralize the blue base in the makeup, creating a soft look." Less sallow skin? Look for yellow-based soft pinks, coral pinks, brownish pinks, rosy-browns, and bronzes.

BLUSH, LIP COLOR FOR BLACK SKIN

"Warm blush colors counteract black skin's tendency to look ashy or gray," says skin and makeup expert Tamara Friedman.

"Avoid too-soft (or light) blush colors, which can look artificial on black skin, and too-dark shades, which can appear muddy. If your skin is light, choose neutral, subtle tones (rather than bright ones) for cheeks. Clear soft coral, soft brick, terra cotta, even a pale-pale red will warm your complexion.

"Medium to dark skin? Look for deep corals, soft browns, dark dusty pinks, or medium shades of burgundy or berry. Colors should be vibrant; the darkness of your skin will tone down most blush colors."

If your skin tone is deep, the dark hue of your lips will soften bright lip colors, so opt for clear, vibrant shades in burgundy, ruby, garnet, deep coral, terra cotta. Lighter skin? Choose subtler colors like soft coral, peach, apricot, rosy-red. Avoid light or frosted lipsticks—they'll contrast too much with dark skin. If your mouth is full, choose matte or semi-matte lip color and skip gloss altogether.

BEAUTY WRAP-UP

1. When applying makeup, play up your best feature. Don't highlight your eyes, cheeks, *and* lips—your makeup will overpower your face.

2. For long-lasting eyeshadow, stroke powder shadow *over* eye pencil or cream shadow.

3. Wear contact lenses? Opt for creamy powder shadow and mascara that's formulated for contact-lens wearers. Avoid "lengthening" mascaras that contain

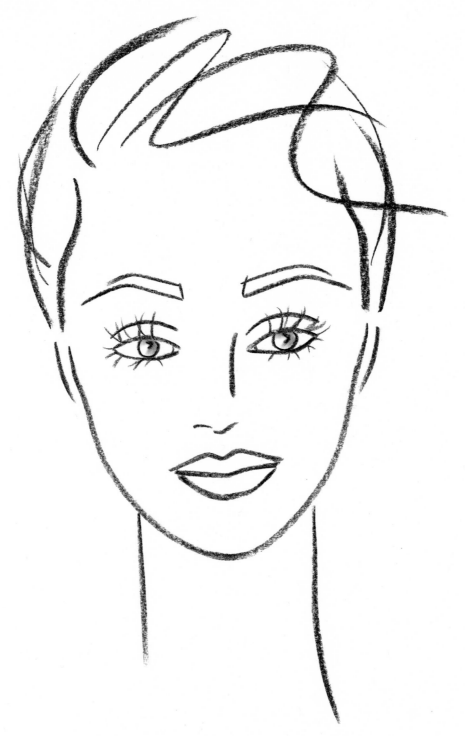

*Use this face chart to sketch your own makeup design
or to practice working with new shades.*

tiny fibers that can get into eyes and cause irritation.

4. If you wear glasses, choose frames that complement your skin and hair shades, flatter your face shape.

5. Dust—don't "paint"—blush color onto cheeks. Keep color subtle, natural.

6. If you have black skin, avoid too-pale or frosted blush colors; they'll look artificial.

7. Asian skin? Experiment with *both* warm and cool colors. Cool cheek and lip shades will give you a soft, feminine look. Warmer tones will provide a natural, subtle beauty.

8. Use a cotton ball or cosmetic puff to blend "edges" of blush into surrounding skin.

9. Don't pair dark liner with pale lipstick. Choose lip liner that matches your lipstick (or opt for one that's "nude").

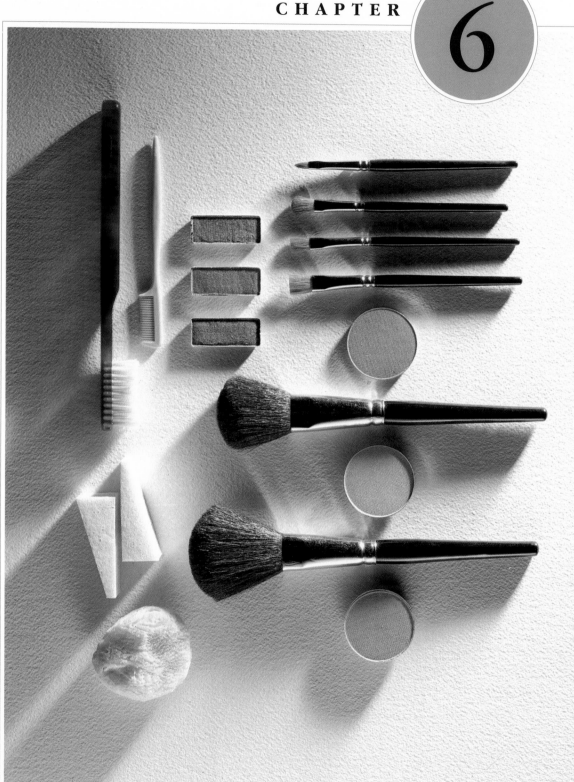

CHAPTER 6

TEN STEPS TO A FABULOUS FACE

1. Smooth moisturizer over face and neck to "prime" skin, allow makeup to go on evenly, stay put.

2. Dab concealer, one shade lighter than skin tone, under eyes (into dark circle), in darker corners of eyes (by nose), and on eyelid (here you can use eyeshadow setting) and blend by patting with fingertip.

3. Dot foundation onto forehead, cheeks, nose, and chin. Blend well, especially around jawline. (Apply with a slightly damp sponge for sheer coverage.)

4. Smooth a hint of foundation over eyelids to keep eye makeup color-true.

5. Using a big, soft brush, dust translucent powder over face and neck.

6. Sweep blush onto "apples" of cheeks, and slightly upward into hairline. Soften "edges" with a cotton ball.

7. Give definition to eyes by lining upper lids; smudge with little fingertip (see "Focus on Eyes," pages 73-74 and "Problem Solvers," page 77, for specific instructions for *your* eye shape). Sweep medium-tone shadow onto lid and into crease. Smooth lighter tone over lids and browbones. Make eyes look larger by accenting outer corners (use a soft pencil or shadow to create little triangles at corners: good color choices include midnight blue, jade, violet, ocean blue, bronze).

8. Apply two coats of smudge-proof, waterproof mascara. Lengthen and thicken lashes by holding mascara wand vertically and sweeping tip back and forth (like a windshield wiper) along ends of lashes. Turn wand to horizontal position and sweep up through lashes, wiggling brush slightly to coat both sides of each lash. Use a lash comb to separate lashes, remove mascara clumps.

9. Fill in sparse brows with brush-on brow powder or a fine-tipped brow pencil in a shade that matches

More Smart Makeup Tricks

99

your hair color. Use a brow comb or brush to "lift" brows (this will "open up" eyes). Tame unruly brows by misting a clean toothbrush or brow brush with hairspray, then lightly comb hairs upward.

10. Apply a lip fixative, then outline lips with pencil that matches your lipstick shade. Smooth on lip color and lightly dust lips with loose powder. Reapply lipstick and gently blot lips with tissue. (Dot gloss onto center of lower lip to make mouth look fuller.)

NIGHTLIGHTS—SPECIAL EFFECTS FOR ROMANTIC EVENINGS

Candlelit rooms call for makeup that catches and reflects light. Colors can be bolder, brighter; eyes and lips should be well-defined. Use a little glitter and gloss here and there for nighttime glow.

· Use eyeliner pencil on lids, below lower lashes to bring out eyes; *don't* smudge lines.

· Add sparkle to eyes with slightly iridescent shadows.

· Highlight cheekbones with a touch of pearlized or frosted blush (dust over matte blush for a natural look).

· Line lips for dimension.

· Opt for moisturizing, rather than matte, lip color, or smooth gloss over your usual matte shade to make lips look shiny, full.

NO MORE MAKEUP MELT-DOWN: THE FADE PROOF FACE

Summer's heat and humidity can melt makeup in a flash. During the colder months, overheated offices and stores can up skin's perspiration and oil output, and makeup can fade away. Here, a guide to making makeup stay put, remain color-true all day.

Oily skin has a hard time "holding onto" makeup, especially foundation and blush. Prep skin by whisking a cotton ball saturated with astringent (one containing alcohol or witch hazel) over oily areas. On drier patches, use a special oil-free moisturizing gel.

Opt for water-based, oil-free, oil-absorbing, or matte foundation. In warmer weather, add a pinch of translucent powder to two fingertips of foundation to create a super-oil-absorbent makeup that will stay color-true.

Always "set" makeup with a light dusting of powder, or pat an oil-absorbent pressed powder over foundation. Powder creates a velvety matte finish, prevents oil breakthrough (and helps keep makeup from "streaking" or wearing away).

If your skin absorbs blusher quickly, use a cream blush, then dust powder blush (in the same color family) over it. Or, dust cheeks with loose powder, stroke on blush, and "set" color with a final dusting of loose powder.

Keep eyeshadow from fading (or accumulating in lid crease) by smoothing a hint of foundation or an eye makeup fixative over lids and browbones. Smooth on powder shadow, then lightly dust lids with loose powder.

Lipstick lasts if you use a lip pencil to outline— then color in—lips. Smooth lipstick (matte shades stay put longer than moisturizing ones) over pencil. Blot with tissue.

Opt for two coats of waterproof, smudge proof mascara. To make sure your eye makeup doesn't smudge, giving you "raccoon" eyes, dip your little finger into loose translucent powder; lightly pat over under-eye area.

SUMMER'S SUN-KISSED LOOK

Come summer, you'll want to make some makeup changes—to give your skin a soft, warm glow.

Almost everyone's skin darkens slightly during the summer, so the foundation that looked so perfect in February may appear pasty by July. Transform your foundation to match your new skin tone by mixing two fingertips of your usual shade of makeup with one fingertip of foundation that's one shade darker.

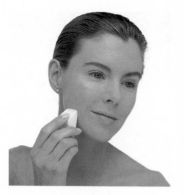

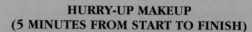

HURRY-UP MAKEUP
(5 MINUTES FROM START TO FINISH)

In a rush? Streamline your morning makeup routine by following these time-saving steps:

30 seconds: Smooth moisturizer over face and neck.

1 minute: Dot concealer under eyes and pat to blend.

1 minute: Using your fingertips or a sponge, dot foundation onto forehead, nose, cheeks, and chin; blend.

1 minute: For natural but well-defined eyes, stroke a neutral eye pencil or eyeshadow along crease in lid and under lower lashes. (Or smudge a pencil onto lids to create illusion of shadow.) (Good color choices: taupe, brown, soft lavender-gray.) Use brow powder to fill in skimpy brows. Stroke on one coat of mascara.

1 minute: Dust loose powder over face; sweep blush onto cheeks.

30 seconds: Smooth a lip fixative onto lips; apply lip color.

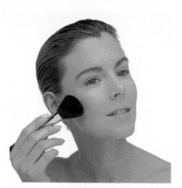

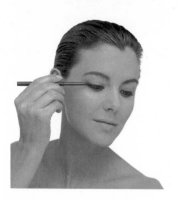

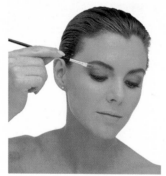

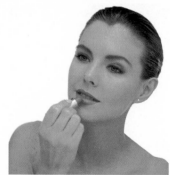

Fair skin? Warm your complexion, creating the illusion of a light golden tan. After applying foundation, dust tawny-peach blushing powder onto cheeks, forehead, nose, chin, shoulders, and breastbone.

Choose warm peachy-apricot or tawny-rose hues for lips, cinnamons, pale rusts, or sea colors like seafoam, muted turquoise, for lids.

102

Dark or olive complexion? Your skin will turn browner during the summer, and earthy colors like taupe and smoky brown will accentuate eyes, while pinky-brown shades will highlight lips, cheeks (opt for a dab of gloss on lower lip).

Black skin does become darker during the summer, so choose (or mix) a sheer foundation one or two shades darker than your usual makeup. Choose neutral, but intense, eye colors like rich cocoa, deep olive, plum. Opt for rosy-brown hues for cheeks and lips.

Want to deepen a light golden tan? Subtly dust cheeks, forehead, nose, chin, shoulders, and breastbone with a medium-toned bronzing powder.

Medium tan skin? Use highlighter to accent temples and cheekbones, and opt for warm, sheer lip color.

SELF-TAN HOW-TO'S

"Faux tans," the kind that come in a bottle, are—according to dermatologists—a good, safe substitute for a real tan. These products are made from dihydroxyacetone, a harmless substance that darkens the outermost layer of the skin, and, used properly, most self-tanning lotions and creams come close to mimicking the real thing. Here are seven steps to a natural-looking golden glow.

1. You'll need to shave and exfoliate your legs (and exfoliate arms, shoulders, face, if you plan to "tan" these areas). Don't use a loofah—you can end up with patchy skin and a streaky tan. Instead, opt for finely milled cleansing grains in a creamy base, and, using a gentle circular motion, massage over legs, arms, shoulders. On your face, slough away dry skin flakes with very fine cleansing grains or a soft complexion sponge.

Shave legs *before* "tanning." If you shave afterward, you'll scrape off parts of your tan.

2. Wait an hour after bathing, exfoliating, and shaving, *then* apply self-tanner. Your skin needs 20 minutes to an hour to recover its natural pH balance, ensuring a more even tan. Prepare skin by smoothing

103

body lotion over areas you're planning to "tan."

3. Smooth self-tanner *evenly* over skin. *Rub in* the product *well*—otherwise, your tan will be spotty. Use less on knees and elbows; this "thicker" skin colors quickly, needs only a minimal amount of tanner.

4. Blend evenly onto feet, on upper thighs, and ask a friend or your partner to evenly spread tanner over your shoulders, back, and neck. Plan to tan your face? Opt for a special self-tanning product formulated for faces, and be sure it's non-comedogenic (doesn't cause acne).

5. Most products tan within three to six hours. To achieve a *darker* color, reapply after three hours.

6. Be sure to wash hands thoroughly after applying, or you could end up with orange palms.

7. You'll need to reapply tanner every three or four days to maintain your golden glow.

(Note: Some self-tan products contain sunscreen, others don't—so be sure to use an SPF 15 sunscreen before any sun exposure.)

BOTTLE-TAN MAKEUP TRICKS

· Most complexions turn a little more red-orange or yellow-orange from self-tanning products than from the sun. To even out a faux tan and make sure it's natural-looking, opt for powder cream makeup or tinted moisturizer one shade darker than your natural skin tone.

· Choose warm, subtle lip and cheek colors—peach, apricot, rosy-brown, soft coral. True pink and clear-red hues can clash with a bottle tan.

COSMETIC COST SAVERS

Mix "Old" Makeups for a New Look

· Apply a soft beige lipstick *under* strong reds, corals, pinks, oranges, fuchsias to soften them.

· If lipstick goes "blue" on lips, apply a gold-toned lip color first to warm up the color.

· Use a light honey-brown loose or pressed powder, or a beige-toned blush over brighter blush shades to tone them down.

· Stroke a pink powder blush over cheeks, then top with a peach blush to achieve a natural tawny, sun-kissed look.

· Use bright blush over a pastel or neutral color to make it more intense, warm, for evening.

· To tone down an intense eyeshadow color, dust a matte taupe or gray heather shadow over it.

· Stroke a shimmery shadow over a matte shadow to transform daytime eye makeup into a glamorous nighttime look.

· Give eyes a smoky look by stroking a matte gray shadow (from light slate to charcoal) over your usual matte shadow. Add a little extra gray shadow to lashline area.

Recycle Almost-Used-Up Makeups

· Mend a broken lipstick by using a match to slightly melt the bottom of the detached piece. Place the two halves together, and heat edges slightly to seal. Cool in refrigerator.

· Just a few drops of foundation left in the bottle? Add a pinch of cornstarch or loose powder, a few drops of water, and blend.

· Salvage an overused cosmetics sponge by soaking it overnight in 1 teaspoon baking soda and a drop of mild dish detergent mixed into 8 ounces warm water.

· Don't discard "down-to-the-rim" lipstick. Use a firm-bristled lipstick brush to pick up color.

·Save old mascara wands. Wash in warm, soapy water to remove color, dry thoroughly, then use to brush brows into place.

HOW TO STRETCH MAKEUP DOLLARS

·Save the paper or plastic inserts that cover powder products. They prevent flaking, which wastes powder.

·Keep cosmetics in a makeup kit, if you carry them in your purse or tote. This will prevent them from getting tossed around, which causes the products to crumble.

·Prevent lipsticks from cracking by extending them no more than 1/2 inch from the tube.

·Don't "pump" a mascara wand. This causes air to enter the tube and dry out the product. Instead, insert wand, twist, and remove.

·Keep cosmetics like lipsticks in the refrigerator during hot weather to prevent melt-down. (Don't leave them in the car on a 90-degree day!)

BEAUTY BLOOPERS

Do's and don'ts for the ten most common makeup mistakes:

1. Don't wear foundation that's too dark for your skin tone; it'll exaggerate fine lines, "pool" in pores, making them look bigger. Do match foundation to skin tone by smoothing a bit onto your jawline (try to test makeup in natural, not fluorescent, light for a perfect match).

2. Don't get caught with a "stripe of blush." Unblended, too-dark blusher will detract from beautiful eyes, make the face appear puffy. Do choose blush shades that complement your skin tone, and dust *lightly* onto "apples" of cheeks (you can always apply more color, if needed). Soften "edges" with translucent powder and puff.

3. Don't draw a harsh lip line, or one that's noticeably darker than your lip color. The line will look fake. Instead, use nude lip liner, or one that matches your lipstick, and draw a soft, subtle line along lip edges. Use a lipstick brush to blend lip color into line.

4. Don't wear super-frosted eyeshadows during the day. They'll emphasize wrinkles and lines in the eye area. Opt for soft matte shades for day, subtly pearlized colors for evening.

5. Don't over- or under-pluck eyebrows. Too-thin brows can look harsh and "age" you. Wild, bushy ones can "weigh down" smaller eyes, making them look even tinier. Stray hairs (especially in the area between the eyes) will give you an unkempt look. Do tweeze brows to remove strays, following the natural arch of the brow. Use muted brow pencil or brush-on brow powder (in a color that matches your hair) to fill in scanty brows.

6. Don't glop on mascara. It'll clump and smudge. Do apply one thin coat at a time and allow to dry between coats (two applications should be sufficient). Use a lash comb to separate lashes, remove mascara clumps.

7. Don't use heavy oil-based foundation in the summer. Even drier complexions will look too shiny. Do opt for sheer moisturizing makeups or water-based foundation for warm-weather wear.

8. Don't use too-light (or white) concealer under eyes. It'll look unnatural—and emphasize dark circles. Do choose concealer that's one shade lighter than your skin tone and pat onto darker areas only, blending well.

9. Don't over-powder your face. Too much powder will cake in fine lines. Do apply loose or pressed powder lightly, then use a cosmetic puff or cotton ball to even and buff.

10. Don't use too-pale or frosted lipstick if you have medium to dark black skin. The contrast will be jarring. Do opt for matte or lightly moisturizing lipsticks that flatter your skin tone.

MAKEUP SHELF LIFE

All cosmetics age over time. Atmospheric or temperature changes can cause ingredient breakdown, and the oil and dirt transferred *from* your skin *to* a particular cosmetic can trigger growth of harmful bacteria or fungi. While lipstick or blush that's past its prime may just look a little dull or off-color on your skin, old *eye makeup* that's contaminated with germs and bacteria can cause serious eye inflammations, including conjunctivitis (an irritation of the eye) and blepharitis (inflammation of the lid). Here, a guide to cosmetic shelf life:

Liquid foundation: Keep one to two years. Discard if it begins to separate (oil on top, clearer liquid on bottom), or doesn't go on evenly, or if you notice a foul odor.

Lipstick: Lasts two to three years. Throw out if you notice beads of oil on the sides or a foul odor.

108

Liquid mascara, eye liners: Replace every three months. (Bacteria and fungi build up quickly on these products—but aren't visible to the naked eye.)

Powder eyeshadow, blush, face powder: Last two to three years. It's wise to replace shadow every year; however, to minimize risk of eye infections throw out products that have started to flake.

BEAUTY SHORTCUTS

1. No time to completely redo makeup before an evening out? Use an astringent pad to remove makeup in T-zone only. Apply liquid (or powder cream) foundation to T-zone. Dust cheeks with a neutral shade of blush. Use tissue to pat away oil from eyelids, and sweep a hint of shadow from lashes up to crease. Tissue off lipstick, smooth a little lip fixative onto lips, and reapply color.

2. Cut your eye makeup application time in half by using a thick-tipped eye pencil in place of liner and shadow. Draw a medium-thick line along lashes. Use fingertip to smudge color upward into crease.

3. No time for mascara? Rub a very soft pencil (blue, brown, muted gray, or plum) onto the tip of your little finger. Smudge color along base of upper lashes, exactly where they emerge from the lids. You'll achieve subtle depth that defines your eyes, gives the appearance of longer lashes.

4. Quickly revive makeup *without* removing foundation by pressing tissue over oily areas of face. Using a powder cream foundation or pressed powder, lightly pat over entire face. Dust blush onto cheekbones.

5. Has foundation started to look a little dull or "flat" on your dry complexion? Renew color and give skin radiance by "spritzing" skin with an atomizer filled with water.

SPECIAL BEAUTY NEEDS FOR THE MOTHER-TO-BE

During pregnancy, an inner radiance shines

through—something perhaps that nature has built in to compensate for a less-than-graceful figure! Whether you feel you have been endowed with this glow or not, you need to be aware of grooming at this time and may need to make temporary alterations in your usual beauty routine. A few points to keep in mind:

· Changes in hormonal balance can affect the complexion. Overactive glands leave some women with acne; others say their skin has never been so clear.

· Your skin may be drier than usual. If so, be sure to use moisturizers best suited for your skin type now.

· If you have facial blemishes, or change in skin pigment, try a sheer or medium-coverage liquid foundation to even out skin tone.

· Brownish stains can develop on the forehead, cheeks, or nose. These are called the "mask of pregnancy." It's mostly found on brunettes, and although there is no way to prevent it, it usually disappears after the baby is born. You can camouflage these marks with a cream or stick concealer in a shade lighter than your own.

· Sometimes increased blood circulation causes too rosy a skin color. Soften with foundation and powder; avoid pink-toned foundations or blush colors.

· If your skin is pale and drab, brighten it up with light, soft tones of blush (powder or cream) and a sheer lipstick in a coordinating tone.

· Eyes can become a focal point by wearing neutral eyeshadow shades and a thin, smudged line of pencil or liquid eyeliner. Avoid heavy eye makeup under the eyes: this will accentuate any darkness or circles under the eyes.

BRIDAL BEAUTY

It's your wedding and you want a special, perfect look. But don't go too far in trying to achieve it—you don't want to appear like a complete stranger walking down the aisle! Remember that you want to look like yourself . . . only better.

Try these suggestions to subtly and attractively enhance your bridal beauty:

1. Have a beauty consultation. Receive makeup advice from a trained professional, and try several different looks before making a final makeup purchase.

2. Tend to your nails! Photographers and friends alike will be studying your ring finger, so start several months in advance with regular manicures to make sure nails are healthy and beautiful. A fresh manicure is a must for your wedding day. Try a soft rosy color, or pick a French manicure for the ultimate in bride elegance.

3. Stay away from orangey makeup colors; they photograph harshly. Stick to shades of rose and mauve, which are lovely against the white and ivory colors of most bridal gowns.

4. Remember, a light dusting of translucent face powder over finished makeup will ensure that makeup stays fresh.

5. Treat yourself to a full set of new makeup brushes for the wedding. Make sure you have selected all natural bristle brushes. You'll enjoy them for many years to come.

6. For long-wearing lipstick: Apply lipstick, blot, apply powder. Apply again, blot, and reapply powder. Apply once more and blot for long-lasting lip color.

7. Buy one shade of lip and nail color for all the bridesmaids so that they look color-coordinated.

8. See a dermatologist if you have a tendency to break out under stress. Begin a regular skin-care regimen to prevent any stress-related skin problems on your wedding day.

9. Have your teeth cleaned.

10. Meet with your hairdresser to discuss your wedding hairstyle. It may be necessary to reshape your current style to meet your wedding hairstyle goal. If

111

your hair is permed, do it now so that it has a good long time to begin to relax. You may also want to discuss reshaping your eyebrows at this time.

11. Have your own "dress rehearsal" to time how long it takes you to get completely ready. That way, you'll avoid rushing at the last minute.

12. Break in your shoes by wearing them for a half hour each day. (Stay on a rug so that they won't scuff.)

CROSS-COUNTRY BEAUTY

Do you live in an area, like *Florida*, that's warm, sometimes humid year 'round? Opt for sheer, not heavy, makeup bases—and choose water-based foundation unless your skin is ultra-dry. Always set foundation with powder to prevent oil breakthrough. Powder eyeshadows are best in these regions.

Skin's at risk for sun-related damage (skin cancer, premature aging) in *Southwestern* states, where the sun shines well into fall and winter. Get everyday protection by using cosmetic products (foundation, eyestick) that contain sunscreen (SPF 8 or higher); or smooth a lightweight SPF 15 sunscreen (choose one formulated for your skin type) onto face before applying makeup.

Windy cities, like *Chicago*, can take a toll on skin that's dry to begin with. Use richer, creamier moisturizer in the winter, allowing it to soak into skin for at least 1 minute, then apply a moisturizing makeup base. Cream-based eyeshadows are a good bet.

BEAUTY WRAP-UP

1. Evening makeup calls for bolder, brighter colors—well-defined lips and eyes.

2. Keep lipstick from wearing off (especially during the summer) by using a lip pencil to "color in" lips, then applying lipstick over pencil.

3. Create the illusion of a tan by using a tawny-peach blush or bronze dusting powder on cheeks, forehead, chin, nose, shoulders, breastbone.

4. If your tan came from a bottle, use "cream pow-

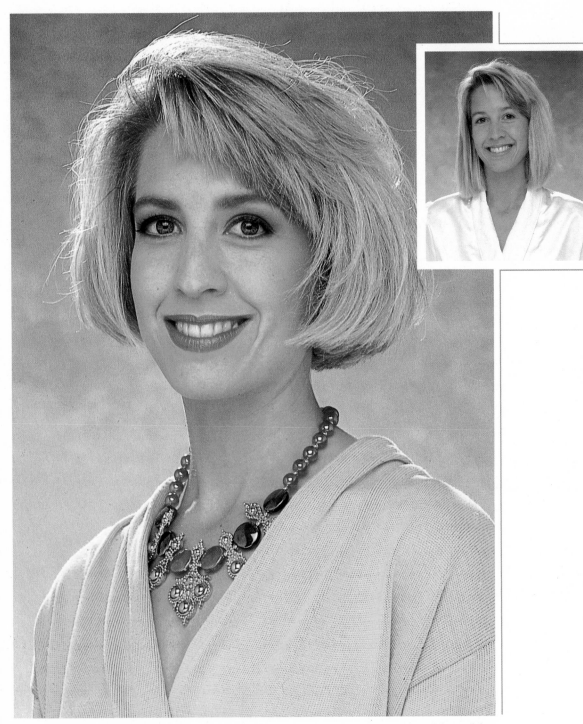

Lisa Vitucci, Temecula, California. *A shorter, fuller hairstyle adds width to Lisa's narrow face and warm cosmetic shades enhance her skin tone. Since Lisa believes that you never look fully dressed without lipstick, a coral lipliner and an apricot lipstick complete her look.*

113

More Smart Makeup Tricks

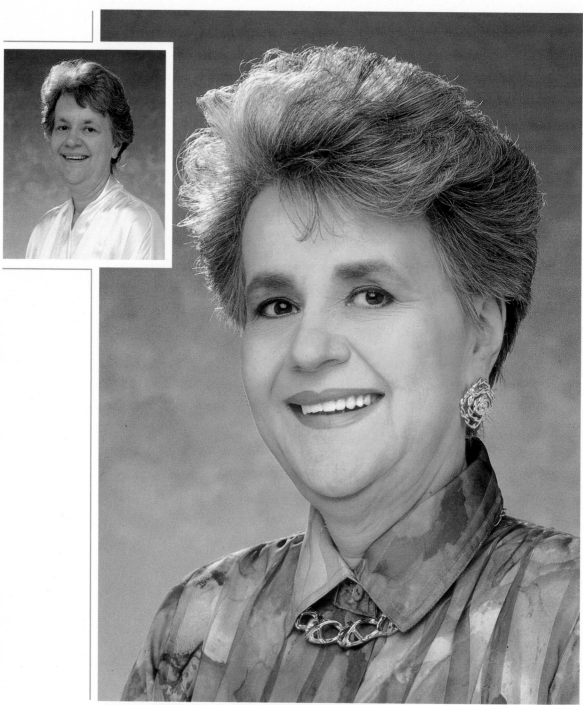

Kay Higginbotham, Shelby, Alabama. *Following a good skin-care regimen has kept Kay's skin in excellent condition. She chooses creamy peach blush to warm her skin tone and soft, neutral makeup shades to complement her brown eyes. Adding height to the crown area of her hairstyle and finishing with bold earrings balance the proportions of Kay's face.*

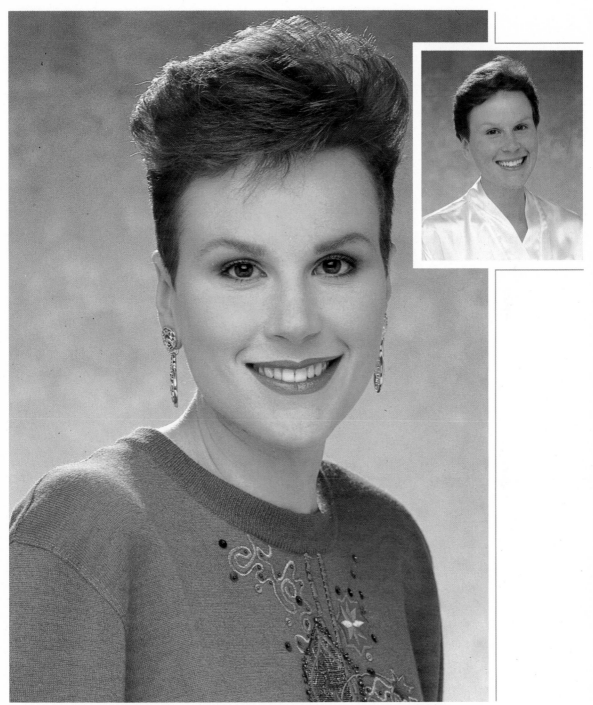

Tara Lundon, Newtown, Pennsylvania*. Brown, copper and teal makeup shades were used to enhance Tara's natural good looks. To emphasize her eyes she dusts her lashes with a fine powder before applying dark brown mascara and uses tawny eyebrow coloring to help frame her eyes. Honey colored blush and mocha lipstick complete her coordinated palette.*

115

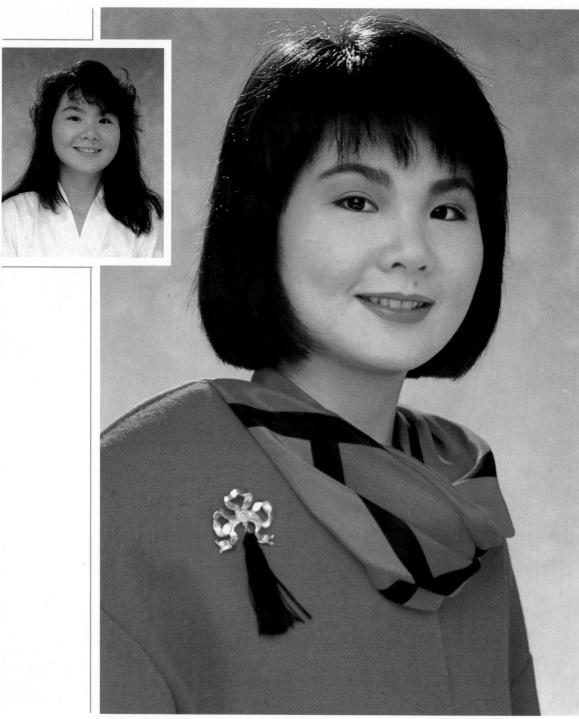

Liana Tse, San Francisco, California. *Liana wears dark brown eyeliner to give her eyes definition and vitality. A warm red lipstick shade adds color to her face and a chin-length haircut with soft bangs makes her face appear more narrow.*

116

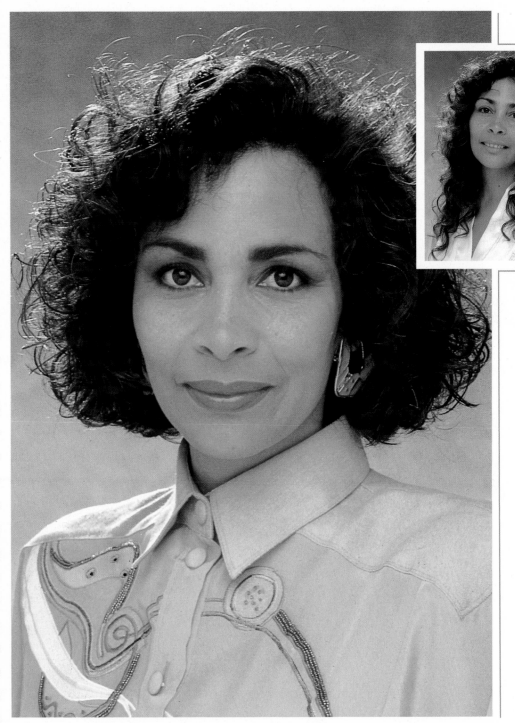

Dolorah Duplessis-Alva, Citrus Height, California. Dolorah's expressive eyes are flattered with bronze, taupe and ginger-toned shadows and black mascara. Rich peach blushing powder complements her olive skin tone, and a fresh, new haircut adds polish to her look.

117

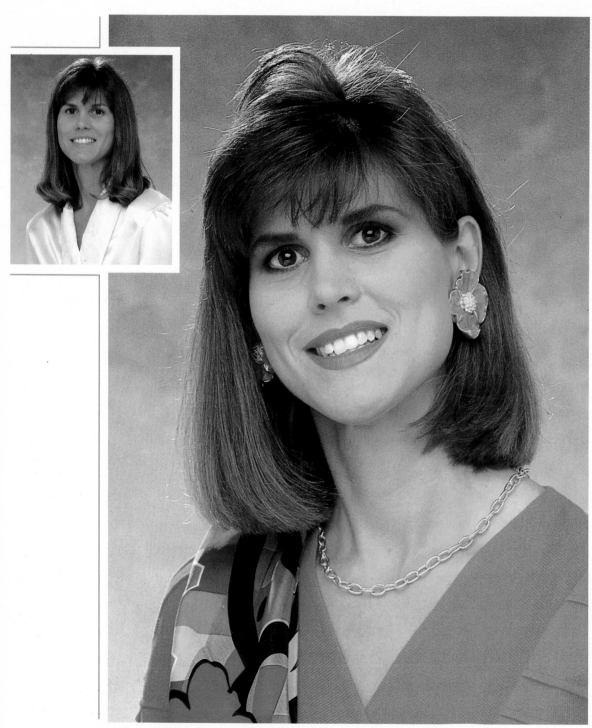

Debra Fritts, Beaverton, Oregon. *A sophisticated, versatile haircut emphasizes Debra's fine features. Heather gray, plum and soft pink eyeshadows define her eyes. Her cheeks and lips are accentuated with rose-pink blush and lipstick.*

118

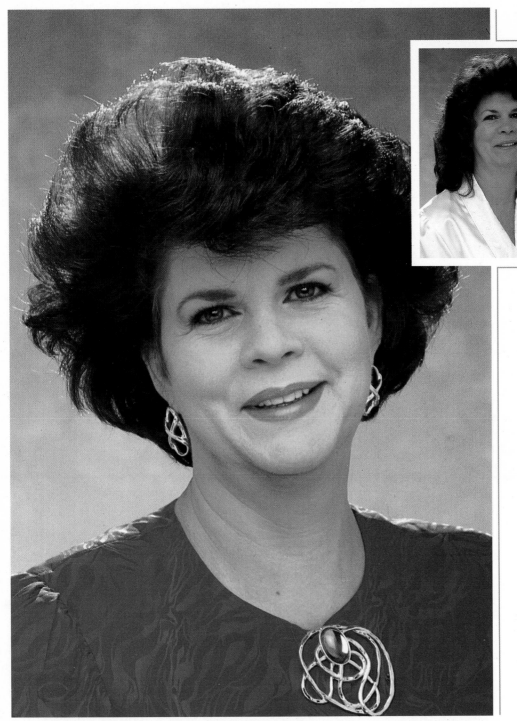

Carolyn Matthews, Florence, South Carolina. *A shorter haircut helps to slenderize Carolyn's face while accentuating her eyes. Violet and opal eyeshadows together with a lining of deep blue accent her eyes and coordinate with her outfit. Lip and cheek colors are raspberry tone.*

119

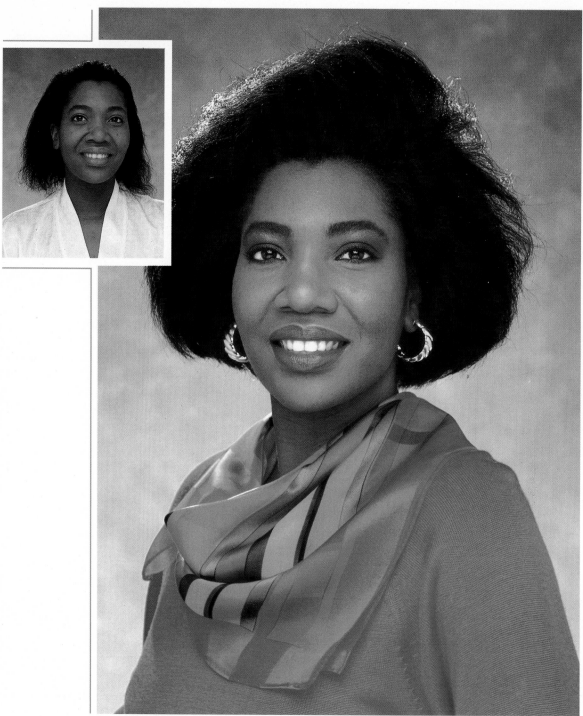

Serilda Foy, Evanston, Illinois. *Deep sable, honey brown and beige eyeshadows blend softly together to play up Serilda's almond-shaped eyes. A spicy red lipstick and scarlet blush accent her wardrobe color. Just a few inches snipped off her hair creates a stylish, face-flattering style.*

der" makeup or a tinted moisturizer to tone down the slightly reddish-orange or yellow-orange hue. Opt for warm, subtle lip and cheek colors in peach, apricot, rosy-brown, or soft coral; nix true pink and clear red colors, which can clash with a bottle tan.

5. Clean your beauty tools (brushes, sponges, puffs) regularly. Applicators can pick up oil from your skin, cause cosmetic colors to change or go on "splotchy."

6. Use a *yellow-based* concealer to minimize purple hue of under-eye circles, and to take the red out of pimples.

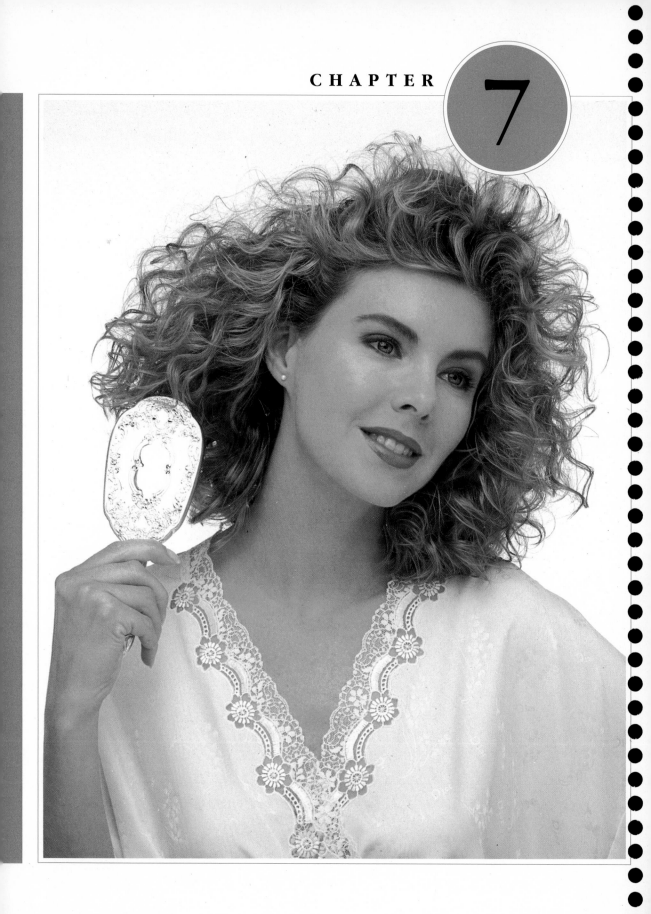

CHAPTER 7

CUTS, CONDITIONING, STYLING

Radiant, healthy hair is a top beauty priority for the majority of women. Hair that's soft and swingy, manageable, and easy to style is an instant confidence and image booster. After all, when your hair looks good, you feel good about yourself (and you project that feeling to others).

Here, a guide to gorgeous hair, starting with guidelines for getting an expert cut that's tailored to your specific hair type, lifestyle, and face shape; a shampooing and conditioning regimen that maximizes the health of your hair; and a host of styling tricks "borrowed" from the top pros.

SALON SENSE

How good your hair looks depends to a great degree on the quality of your salon's staff. Top-notch stylists can literally "cut" body into fine, thin hair. Skilled colorists can make dull, drab hair vibrant, glossy. Perming pros can turn limp locks into voluminous waves. But finding a salon that meets all your hair-care needs (while minimizing the chances of "hair disasters"—like the too-short cut, carrot-red dye job, or frizzy perm) takes a little know-how. Rick Garcia, owner of the Rick Garcia Salon, in Westport, Connecticut, tells how to scout out the best salon and stylist.

When you see someone who's got a great cut, don't hesitate to ask for the name of her salon and stylist. (You may need to approach a perfect stranger at a mall, or on the street—but be assured that most people are tremendously flattered when complimented on their haircut!)

If you've heard that a particular salon is good, but need to know which stylist can give you the best cut, ask the salon manager or receptionist to recommend a stylist who specializes in cutting *your type of hair.*

Great-Looking Hair

123

(Some stylists excel at blunt cuts; others specialize in cutting short, curly hair.)

Before booking an appointment for a cut, color, or perm, call the salon and ask for a complimentary consultation. The stylist can examine your hair and recommend styles (or coloring or perming processes) that are right for you (some stylists prefer to set aside 30 to 40 minutes for a consultation; that way, if the client decides then and there to go ahead with a cut or quick coloring procedure, she can).

When you arrive at the salon do a "head check." Do other clients walk away with good cuts, color, and perms? How quickly do clients move from the waiting area to shampoo sinks to styling chairs? If the waiting room is jam-packed with women nervously glancing at their watches, chances are the salon is more interested in quantity than quality.

Do a cleanliness survey as well. Is the salon immaculate, with well-swept floors, clean sinks, sterilized equipment? (Cutters should have comb and brush sanitizers at each station.)

To get the best cut for your lifestyle and looks ask the stylist, "How do you perceive me?" In choosing the perfect cut for you, the stylist will take into account the condition and texture of your hair, your facial shape, *and* your body shape. A good stylist will view you as a total package, not just a head of hair that needs cutting. He will probably also ask about your occupation, family responsibilities, and how much time you have to spend on your hair each day.

After your stylist has recommended a certain cut, feel free to show him pictures of cuts you've clipped from magazines. But be open-minded: the short boy cut you love may not work for your face shape or hair texture.

Prevent haircut disasters by making sure you understand exactly what your stylist has in mind—and by explaining what you definitely *don't* want. Many women complain they went in for a trim and walked out with a full-fledged cut. If you're afraid the stylist might snip off too much hair, say, "I'd like to keep my hair on the long side," or "I *only* need a trim." (Remember that hair grows approximately half an inch each month.)

If you're unhappy with a cut (or color or perm), should you ask that your hair be restyled or reprocessed? Or should you go to another salon? A stylist may need to cut your hair once or twice before getting a "feel" for it and achieving the perfect cut. Give him the benefit of the doubt—but if the third cut isn't what you want, switch to another stylist. If you're *very* unhappy with a cut, color, or perm, ask that the work be redone. Most salons stand behind their work and want to please clients.

What if you have been loyal to your stylist for years—but long to have another person at the *same* salon cut your hair? Talk with your long-time stylist and diplomatically explain that you'd like a new look, a cut you've noticed the other stylist giving his or her clients.

Chances are your regular stylist will suggest you switch to his colleague. After many years of cutting someone's hair, a stylist can "burn out." He may realize that another cutter will have a fresh perspective on the client's hair.

Don't trim your bangs at home in between cuts. You'll risk destroying the line of the cut. Many salons offer a complimentary bang trim. Others may charge from $5 to $10 to shape bangs.

TIPPING

Confused as to how much to tip the various staff members at your salon?

Stylists: 10 to 15 percent of the cost of the cut.

Colorists: 10 to 20 percent of cost of process, depending on how much work has been done.

Shampoo person: $1 to $2.

Person who does blow-dry: 10 percent of cost of blow-dry, or $2 to $4 if stylist cost is included in price of cut.

Person who does your perm: 15 to 20 percent of cost of perm.

Perming assistant: $3 to $5, depending on how much work she does.

(Note: There's no need to tip the salon owner if he or she does your cut, color, or perm. But do tip the salon manager for services rendered.)

ASIAN HAIR—CUT WITH CARE

The popular notion that all Asian women are born with thick, straight, coarse hair is a myth. "Actually,

Asian women can have strong, straight hair or fine curly hair, and everything in between," says Yosh, owner of the Yosh For Hair salons in San Francisco and Palo Alto, California.

The success of a cut depends on how well your stylist understands your hair, notes Yosh. "The cutter should always work with, or cut with—not against—the natural direction or movement of the hair (particularly if the hair is coarse)," he cautions. If your stylist cuts against the natural direction, you can end up with hair that springs out wildly in places and is hard to control.

Need to use gobs of gel (or lots of spray) to keep your hair in place? "You've got the wrong cut for your hair type!" notes Yosh.

> · A great cut is the key to a successful hairstyle.
>
> · Your hairstyle should suit your age, lifestyle, and personality—*and* flatter your face and body shapes.
>
> · Elaborate hairstyles that require a lot of upkeep aren't practical for on-the-go women. Opt for a simple, easy-to-manage style.
>
> · "Big" hair can overpower a small person. Closely cropped hair can make a larger women's head look too small for her body.

AFRICAN-AMERICAN HAIR

African-American women are fortunate to have hair that shapes and conforms to most cuts easily and can be "molded" into shape. Because of this, there's no need for excessive use of sprays, gels, or mousses.

Your hairline may tend to be fragile and in many cases much breakage occurs here. (Be especially careful of excessive curling-iron work.)

If you're considering a one-length style and are thinking about chemical straightening, consult with your stylist. These straightenings should be done very, very carefully to prevent breaking and splitting. Be sure the stylist is experienced with the process—it takes a long time to recover from a bad straightening.

FACE-SHAPERS

"The right hairstyle will flatter your facial shape, minimizing any 'beauty flaws,'" says styling pro Rick Garcia. "The wrong style," he adds, "will emphasize certain problems, so it's essential that you and your stylist take your face's shape into consideration before he begins to cut." Here is Garcia's guide to cuts that flatter the six basic face shapes:

Oval Face (slightly narrower at jawline than at temples).

Do's: To enhance your perfect oval face, focus attention on the temples and around the ear areas for balance, keeping hair fullest at the widest part of your face.

Don'ts: None! You have the ideal face shape—and can carry off almost any style.

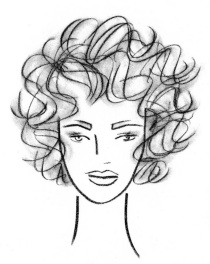

OBLONG

Oblong Face (long, slender, with equal widths at forehead and just below cheekbones; may have narrow or pointed chin).

Do's: If you have a high forehead, minimize the length and width—with soft bangs and a side part. To "widen" a narrow chin, choose a short or medium-length style with fullness in the nape area.

Don'ts: Avoid too much height in the crown area, which can "lengthen" your face. Steer clear of short-short boy cuts featuring a "clean" or bare neck—they'll make your chin look "pointy." Don't comb hair away from your forehead; again, you'll add length to your face.

Round Face (full, round, with rounded chin—widest point is at cheeks and ears).

Do's: If your hair is medium-length to long, bring it forward onto the face to create a more "oval" appearance. Opt for height at the crown to "lengthen" the face. For shorter hair, begin creating height near the temples and up into the crown.

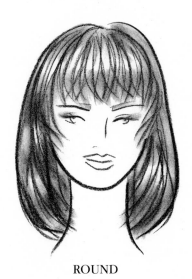

ROUND

127

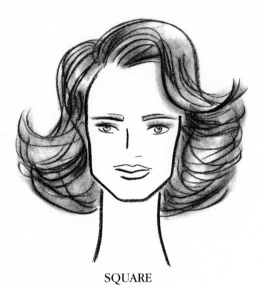

SQUARE

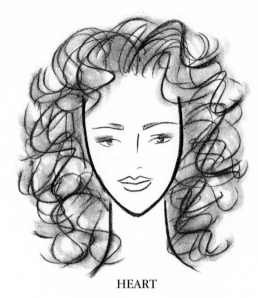

HEART

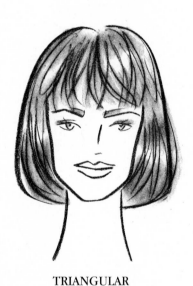

TRIANGULAR

Don'ts: Avoid wearing hair brushed back, which can highlight the roundness.

Square Face (strong, square jawline).

Do's: A square face is a beauty plus, showing strength. You can be creative, experimenting with various styles—and depending on your body shape, you can go with long *or* short locks—and brush or pull hair back from your face to accent the shape.

Don'ts: Avoid the temptation to soften the geometric lines of your face—you'll play down, rather than enhance, your natural beauty.

Heart-Shape Face (wide at temples, narrowing gradually to a small chin).

Do's: You'll need to do a little "camouflaging," creating soft side bangs at the temples to minimize the width. Longer hair with fluffiness or fullness in the chin area will "widen" a narrow chin. (Curly hair works well to reproportion a heart-shaped face.)

Don'ts: Avoid shorter styles, which will accentuate the heart shape, call attention to a "pointy" chin.

Triangular Face (strong jawline, narrowing to a slightly pointed chin; narrowing just a little upward in cheek and temple areas).

Do's: Keep hair close to face, covering the widest

128

part of the temple areas. Opt for a little height at the crown (but not too much!) to break the triangle effect.

Don'ts: Avoid off-the-face styles, which will emphasize the geometric lines of your face's shape. If your hair is straight, don't tuck it behind your ears—you'll call attention to the widest areas. Avoid too much fullness at the jawline.

MORE FACE-FLATTERING TIPS

High forehead: Opt for bangs or a side part to minimize length.

Low forehead: Create the illusion of length by combing hair away from the face. If you prefer the look of bangs, make sure they're light, wispy.

Short neck: Opt for shorter hair with height at the crown to make your neck appear longer.

Large nose: A full hairstyle, with fluffy bangs, will detract from your prominent nose.

Receding chinline: Comb hair forward onto cheeks.

Prominent chinline: Balance by wearing hair high on top, fuller at sides.

Double chin: Camouflage by wearing hair in a modified pageboy, with shorter sides and longer, fuller back, or flip ends upward.

Long neck: Rejoice! You can wear short, medium, or long styles—anything that plays up this beautiful feature.

Glasses wearers: Keep hair smooth, soft—a pretty frame for your face.

HEALTHY HAIR HOW-TO'S

Shiny, silky hair is determined in part by heredity. Some of us were blessed at birth with thick, strong hair; others ended up with fine, fragile locks. But how you care for your hair can play a major role in getting and keeping it super-healthy and radiant. Thanks to recent advances in hair-care technology, you can choose shampoos and conditioners tailored to meet your hair's particular needs.

Wash 'n' Wear

Most shampoos and conditioners today are marked for the type of hair they're meant for. Select the product compatible with your hair type and hair condition.

If you have shampoo or conditioner at home that you're currently using and it's not doing the job, finish it—you've probably spent good money on it. (Or use it on your pet; chances are he won't complain!) Don't accumulate products or try to mix one with another to develop the "right" mix. (For instance, use shampoos and conditioners from the same product line. They've been formulated to work together.)

Remember to seek products clearly marked for your hair type. You might want to try sample sizes of a product if they're available or buy the smaller size products until you find one right for you. Ask your hairstylist to direct you to the product best for your hair.

If your hair is fine, limp, or oily, look for products containing protein or balsam to add body. Avoid cleansing with very warm water—you'll overstimulate your already active sebaceous glands and end up with greasy locks halfway through the day. Instead, use barely lukewarm water. Apply a light protein or silicone-based conditioner to ends of hair only. (Silicones lubricate hair well, won't cause "hair droop.")

Rinse hair *at least* 60 seconds to remove all shampoo/conditioner residue, and follow with a cold-water rinse to smooth the cuticle on the hair shaft, and give hair shine.

Twice a month, deep condition your hair, using a protein-based treatment. Work evenly through the hair, starting at ends and massaging halfway up hair shaft. Leave in for 3 to 5 minutes, then rinse well. (Try a vinegar rinse to curb oiliness, leave hair shiny and manageable: mix 1 teaspoon apple cider vinegar in 8 ounces cold water; pour through hair, then rinse well with cool water.)

If your hair is dry, chemically processed, or frequently exposed to chlorine or salt water, opt for shampoos and conditioners formulated for dry or damaged hair (some incorporate the word "remois-

130

turizing" in the name). Use a 60-second remoisturizing conditioner (cream rinse) after every shampoo, working the product into the entire length of the hair, from roots to ends. Once a week, use an intensive deep remoisturizing cream or conditioner. Hot-oil treatments can temporarily restore shine to extremely dry or dull hair. Leave on for 10 to 15 minutes.

If your hair is "virgin"—unprocessed and in good shape—"cleansing" or "clarifying" shampoos that don't leave any residue, but do remove leftover styling sprays, gels, and mousses, are a best bet for your hair type. Use a very light protein lotion conditioner after shampooing, applying to ends only. Leave in 10 to 20 seconds maximum to prevent overconditioning. Apply a 60-second remoisturizing cream, working product from ends halfway up the length of hair. Leave on for 2 to 3 minutes maximum.

Black women need to pay special attention to shampooing and conditioning. Your hair can be fragile—and on the dry side. What's more, because it's curly, it doesn't catch and reflect light the way straight hair does, so you'll need to condition it regularly in order to flatten the cuticle of individual hairs, and boost shine.

Choose shampoos and conditioners that are formulated to "remoisturize dry or damaged hair." (If your hair is chemically straightened or color-treated, look for products formulated for processed hair.) Rinse scrupulously after shampooing and conditioning—your hair is porous and will "grab onto" dulling residue. Use a cream rinse after every shampoo, and when needed, deep condition with a hot-oil treatment or an intensive remoisturizing cream.

After blow-drying, work a dab—a dime's worth—of a glossy finish, or a dab of hairdressing or pomade, through hair to bring a sheen to it.

Asian hair is often stick straight—and straight hair gets oily faster than curly locks (that's because the oil can travel rapidly down the hair shaft). "Cleansing" shampoos are preferable to moisturizing or body-building ones, which can leave a dull film on your hair.

Asian hair is generally very strong and healthy and needs minimal conditioning. Use a protein-based lotion after every shampoo, applying to ends only, or

---

The Low-down on pH

You may want to test the pH balance of various shampoos and conditioners to find the ones that work best on your hair. (You can quickly test the pH factor of any product by using litmus paper, available at most drugstores.)

The pH factor of a shampoo or conditioner indicates the degree of acidity or alkalinity in the product. A pH rating in the 4 to 8 range tells you the product is "balanced."

Products with a low pH factor (2 to 4) are more acidic, smoothing the cracked cuticle on dry or damaged hair. Shampoos and conditioners with a higher pH factor (7 or above) are quite alkaline and can gently "rough up" the cuticle on oily, limp hair, making it seem thicker, giving it more body. A rating of 11 or higher signals danger—the product could dissolve your hair!

working from tips halfway up length of hair. Leave in 10 to 20 seconds. Once every few weeks, deep condition with a remoisturizing cream; leave in for 5 minutes.

SHAMPOO (AND CONDITIONING) SAVVY

1. Gently brush your hair to loosen dandruff particles, distribute oils, get rid of falling hairs.

2. Using comfortably warm water, thoroughly wet hair before applying shampoo.

3. Pour a minimal amount—about a "quarter's worth"—of shampoo into your wet palms and rub hands together to work up lather. Gently massage shampoo into scalp and "stroke" through hair (don't *rub* hair—you'll risk tangling and breakage). If you're trying to remove a lot of styling-aid residue, don't add more shampoo—you won't be able to effectively rinse it out. Instead, rinse hair for 30 seconds, then re-wash with a "nickel's worth" of shampoo.

4. Rinse hair thoroughly.

5. If your hair is fine or oily, apply conditioner to ends only.

6. For normal or dry hair, work in conditioner *evenly* throughout. Avoid globbing it onto outer hair only—you'll end up with hair that's overconditioned and limp in some areas, underconditioned and flyaway in others.

7. Rinse hair *at least* 60 seconds after conditioning to remove residue, especially if your hair is oily,

limp, permed, or color-treated (processed hair absorbs conditioner quickly, "hangs onto" it).

8. Always finish with a cold-water rinse to smooth and seal the hair's cuticle and promote shine.

9. Blot (don't rub) dry with a big towel.

SHINE-STOPPERS: HOW TO PREVENT HAIR ABUSE

Over-styling: Used properly, blow-dryers won't harm your hair, but all too often, women find their hair is dull, dry—even breaking off—because of blow-dryer abuse! To prevent heat damage, allow your hair to air-dry for 5 to 10 minutes before styling. Then, holding dryer 6 to 8 inches from your head, move it rapidly back and forth (avoid blasting hot air at any one area for too long). Use a warm setting for a minute or so, until moisture begins to evaporate. Then switch to a cool setting.

Over-curling: If you use hot rollers or a curling iron every day, you're courting eventual damage (you can even burn hair with some appliances!). Limit hot roller use to two or three times a week. (To really guard against splitting or breakage and when time permits, wrap tips of hair in end papers, available at drugstores). Use rollers that are warm, not hot-hot, and leave in for a max of 15 minutes. Use curling irons cautiously: heat to warm, not hot, and leave in for a few seconds only. Otherwise, you can end up with crimped, frizzy hair and split ends.

Prime and protect hair with a spray-on setting lotion/conditioner designed to guard against damage from heat appliances.

Over-gooping: Mousses, gels, sprays—all can give your hair body, direction, and control. But used too often, or layered one over the other, they can coat hair with a dulling buildup. Opt for alcohol-free mousses and gels whenever possible (they won't dry your hair as much as alcohol-based products). Also, use styling aids that contain conditioners to boost shine.

Choose lightweight hairsprays that hold hair gently, rather than products that mold hair into a stiff "helmet" (avoid sprays containing lacquer).

When combing hair that has been styled with sprays, gels, mousses, and spritzes, use a wide-tooth comb and begin detangling at the ends of the hair (work your way gradually up to roots).

SUMMERPROOF HAIR

Too much fun in the sun (and salt water and chlorinated pools) can wreak havoc with even the healthiest hair, leaving it dry and dull.

Here are eight steps to summerproof hair:

1. The sun's ultraviolet (UV) rays can damage hair, making it dry and lackluster. UV rays can also cause highlighted hair to turn brassy; color-treated hair to take on a reddish tinge. While shampoos and conditioners containing sunscreen offer *some* protection, your best bets are leave-in products, such as mousses, gels, setting lotions, and sprays that contain sunscreens (look for ones with an SPF of 6 or higher). Note: If you're sensitive to PABA, a sunscreen chemical that can trigger rashes, redness, and itching in a few people, check hair product labels carefully. Many contain PABA.

Highlighted or color-treated hair? Keep color from turning by wearing a hat or scarf.

2. Chlorine and salt water can dry out hair, leaving it straw-like, hard to manage. What's more, chlorine can turn highlighted or bleached hair *green*, give tinted hair a greenish cast, and turn red-tinted hair muddy brown (chlorine can also rob *natural* color from hair, leaving it faded).

Protect your hair from salt and chlorine by massaging a heavy cream conditioner (look for one that contains sunscreen) into hair, from roots to ends. Or work an SPF 15 waterproof sunscreen (the kind you use on your body!) through your hair. Use lots of either product—you want to create a waterproof barrier. Reapply as needed.

3. If you have highlighted or color-treated hair, give it double protection by combing 1 teaspoon of conditioner from roots to ends, then don a snug-fitting

134

swim cap. (Yes, a swim cap—they're back and available in terrific colors to coordinate with all your swim wear.)

4. After swimming, use a cleansing shampoo, or one formulated for swimmers, to wash away conditioner, sunscreen, or oil, plus any traces of salt or chlorine. Follow with a conditioner suited to your particular hair type.

5. A super chlorine- and salt-removing wash? Mix equal parts cleansing shampoo and club soda. The effervescent action of the soda will penetrate the cuticle to "bubble out" residue!

6. African-American hair dries out quickly and can easily break after repeated exposure to sun, salt water, or chlorine. Follow all the above suggestions, *and* work an SPF 15 leave-in conditioner through hair before any lengthy exposure to sun. Try to cut back on blow-drying during the summer months. Air-dry hair whenever possible, or use a moisturizing cream on hair *before* blow-drying.

7. Have hair cut every 4 to 6 weeks (hair grows faster during warmer months) to snip away split ends. Whatever your hair type, deep condition once a week to protect hair's elasticity, and give hair polish.

8. Don't pull wet hair tightly back into a ponytail or chignon. Wet hair "shrinks" as it dries, and you'll risk breakage.

COLD COMFORT FOR WINTER-DRY HAIR

While summer takes the greatest toll on hair, winter can pose a slew of problems too. Follow these quick and easy suggestions for winterproofing your hair:

Unless you live in a damp climate (like the Seattle area), your hair will lose lots of moisture during the winter, ending up dry and flyaway; because it lacks the elasticity that moisture provides, it'll be low on volume. To add moisture to your environment—and your hair—use humidifiers in the living room and bedroom, and, if possible, at your office. Keep home temps in the 68-degree area.

Over-heated rooms can dry hair and rob it of shine. You'll need to condition more frequently—even change products. If you have oily hair and normally use a light protein lotion after shampooing, switch to a light cream remoisturizing product, or alternate the two. Dry or damaged hair? Switch from a 60-second remoisturizing cream to an intensive deep-treatment product—but leave it on hair for 1 minute only, instead of the 5 to 15 minutes recommended on the package.

Protect hair from winds, which can dry it out and cause tangling, by wearing a hat or scarf made of natural fibers. Choose wool hats or scarves or silk scarves; both will help keep you warm. *Avoid* acrylic or acrylic-lined hats—they'll leave hair full of static. To prevent hat-flat hair, steer clear of snug-fitting caps. Instead, use big, over-sized wool berets (roll long hair around your hand and tuck up into hat), or wool hoods that fit loosely. Cold ears? Wear earmuffs *under* the hood.

Hair still flat after taking off your hat? Bend over and mist underneath hair lightly with a low-alcohol hairspray; flip head up and spritz top hairs to help prevent flyaways. (For added volume, gently tease underneath hair before spraying.)

Prevent hair that stands on end by misting the insides of hats and hoods with a spray-on static minimizer (available at drug and variety stores).

Use a natural bristle brush and wooden comb; they'll trigger fewer static attacks than plastic tools.

Quickly smooth flyaway hair by misting a brush with spray, then lightly running it over top hairs. Or, moisten hands with water; rub a tiny amount of gel, hand lotion, leave-in conditioner, or facial moisturizer into palms. Lightly pat hands over hair.

Consider color for a quick mid-winter lift. Winter-dry locks can look dull, faded, and highlights or semi-permanent color (look for one that conditions) can give hair super shine and richness.

If hair is drooping because cold temperatures, winds, have robbed it of elasticity—and body—opt for a gentle body wave to add bounce.

Brush hair very lightly every night—about 15 strokes—to distribute oil from roots to ends, lock in moisture. (Use a natural bristle brush.)

HAIR BOOSTERS

Mother nature may have given you fine, limp hair—or a head full of frizzies—but there's no need to live with hair that's unmanageable, thanks to the dozens of "hair helpers" on the market. However, choosing the right product for your hair type (and hair problems) can be tricky. Should you use a gel to give your fine hair body—or a mousse? What's the difference between a spritz and a spray? A leave-in conditioner and a hairdressing? Here, a mistakeproof guide:

Gels are best for thick, coarse, or medium-textured curly hair, giving it direction and hold. (Avoid using gels on fine hair—they'll weigh it down. You *can* use a tiny dab of gel to softly "mold," control fine bangs that tend to flop, however.) Work gel through damp or dry hair and use your fingers to give your hair direction. (Use a "dime's worth" on short hair, a "nickel's worth" for medium lengths, and a "quarter's worth" for long hair.)

Liquid or *spray gels* work well on most hair types (even finer locks) and are lighter than regular gels. They also give you more control, since you can apply them precisely where you need hold. Use on damp or dry hair.

Mousses boost volume and provide hold for fine, limp hair by "swelling" the hair shaft and making hair appear thicker. Rub a pouf of mousse into palms of hands, then work lightly through roots of damp hair (don't apply to length of hair—you'll end up with sticky, droopy tresses). Use about a "half dollar's worth" of mousse for short and medium-length hair. For long hair, a palmful. Style by blow-drying, or allow hair to air-dry as you "finger scrunch" hair into place.

Spritzes are similar to hairsprays, but hold better and longer. Use on fine and medium-textured dried hair for spot styling—like giving lift and hold to bangs.

Styling sprays (setting lotions) are terrific for fine hair, providing volume and hold. Use a minimal amount on damp hair before blow-drying.

Leave-in conditioners provide condition, gloss, and control for thick, curly styles (and they help prevent frizzies in humid weather, smooth split ends). A good option for coarse or thick hair.

Pomades are a heavier version of leave-in conditioners, providing shine and moisture. Best used on surface hairs only (rub a dab the size of a pea between palms and smooth lightly over dry hair). Ideal for African-American hair and thick, coarse, curly locks.

Hairdressings are lighter than pomades, but heavier than leave-in conditioners, providing shine, moisture, and some direction. Use sparingly—a "pea's worth" at most—and work through dry hair or smooth over top hairs.

Hairsprays give overall hold. For best results, opt for lighter sprays and mist underneath hairs as well as top hair to prevent a "hairspray helmet" that will eventually weigh down locks.

Polishers (or laminates or glazes) provide soft hold and super gloss. Most contain little or no water and rely on silicones to give hair shine without weighing it down. Silicones also form a super *moisture barrier* on the hair—keeping it from drooping or frizzing in humid weather. Can be used on any type of hair, but work best on medium to long, straight, sleek styles. Available in liquid and gel forms.

SMART STYLING TRICKS

Styling gels can leave hair dull, dry—and, in some cases, stiff-looking. If you use gel every day, dilute it with a drop of water or a dab of leave-in conditioner. Your hair will look shinier and feel softer.

To give fine, limp hair maximum lift at the roots, try this styling technique: Use a round bristle brush to lift sections of hair upward. Mist roots with spray gel or a light hairspray. Aim nozzle of dryer at roots for a few seconds; allow hair to cool, then dry entire length.

Give blunt-cut hair extra oomph with this post-styling technique: Flip head forward and mist underneath hair with a light spray. Blow-dry (use cool setting) for several seconds. Flip head up and use a brush or comb to smooth top hairs.

Keep stray hairs (and flyaways) from spoiling a pulled-back style by misting a cotton ball with firm-hold hairspray and running it lightly over hair.

If gel won't keep your bangs from flopping, mold them into place by spritzing a firm-hold hairspray onto tips of index finger and thumb. Quickly work through bangs to shape (they'll stay put all day).

Whether you use hot rollers, regular rollers, a curling iron, or a blow-dryer and round brush, keep just-curled hair from unfurling by allowing curls to *cool completely* before you brush or comb hair.

BEAUTY SHORTCUTS

Problem: Your hair is limp (or greasy) and there's no time to rewash and restyle it before an important party.

Solution: Use a dab of gel to slick back sides (tuck them behind your ears) and lift, then pull bangs forward. Mist lightly with spray, and complement this sophisticated style with eye-catching earrings.

Problem: Your all-one-length hair is drooping because you've overconditioned it.

Solution: Flip head forward and mist underneath hair with spray. Flip head back up and mist top hairs. Gently run a natural bristle brush through hair. The alcohol in the hairspray will absorb the oily residue from the conditioner, and give your hair more volume. (You can also try a hair band or terrific hair accessory to pull hair back.)

Problem: You styled your hair with mousse, gel, or spray in the morning, but by midday (or evening) it's sagging.

Solution: Don't restyle by gooping on more mousse, gel, or spray. Instead, simply moisten your fingers with water and run them through your hair (or lightly mist hair with H_2O) to fluff and restyle locks, or slick them back. Water reactivates most styling products.

Problem: Your bangs are growing out—and flopping onto your face. How can you conceal them?

Solution: Comb a firm-hold gel into wet bangs, then use a flat natural bristle brush to smooth them back, blending them into rest of hair. Allow bangs to air-dry and "mold" into place.

Problem: You wake up late—and there's no time to wash and style your hair.

Solution: Rely on a wide, stretchy sixties-style headband to conceal the oiliest areas and to cover cowlicks. Pull the band down to the hairline (it'll cover a major area of your crown and sides of head) and clip on a pair of spectacular earrings.

CROSS-COUNTRY BEAUTY

Live in the *Northeast?* Your hairstyle will have to stand up to nonstop heat and humidity during the summer months. Keep curly hair from kinking by mixing a dab of gel with a dot of any hairdressing or leave-in conditioner. Work lightly through damp or just-dried locks.

Southwesterners know that the sun shines almost all year 'round and UV rays can damage hair even during the winter. Protect your hair with leave-in products—mousses, hairsprays, gels—that contain sunscreens. Color-treated hair? Be sure to wear a hat or scarf to keep hair from turning brassy or reddish.

If you're from the *Midwest*, you know that cold temperatures, 50-mile-an-hour winds can rob your hair of moisture, leaving it dry and faded. Use an intensive remoisturizing treatment when needed to restore shine, elasticity. Protect hair with a scarf or hat whenever you're outdoors. Consider a combination semi-permanent conditioning/coloring product to add gloss, richness to winter-parched hair.

Many areas of the *Pacific Northwest* are damp and drizzly from November through May. Keep fine hair from drooping by using a firm-hold mousse. Curly hair? Choose a gel mixed with a dot of leave-in conditioner.

BEAUTY WRAP-UP

1. Choose the right shampoo and conditioner for your hair type—the wrong products can either dry out hair, or leave it limp and lifeless.

140

2. Don't be guilty of hair abuse: Use blow-dryers on the lowest setting, holding the nozzle 6 to 8 inches from your hair—and avoid blasting hot air at any one area for too long. Limit hot roller and curling iron use to two or three times a week.

3. Protect hair (especially African-American hair, which tends to be fragile and brittle) from the sun's harmful rays. Use mousse, gel, or spray with an SPF 6 to 15.

4. Winterproof your hair by stepping up your conditioning regimen. Cold temperature, strong winds, overheated rooms—all rob hair of moisture, shine, color, and body. Deep condition frequently.

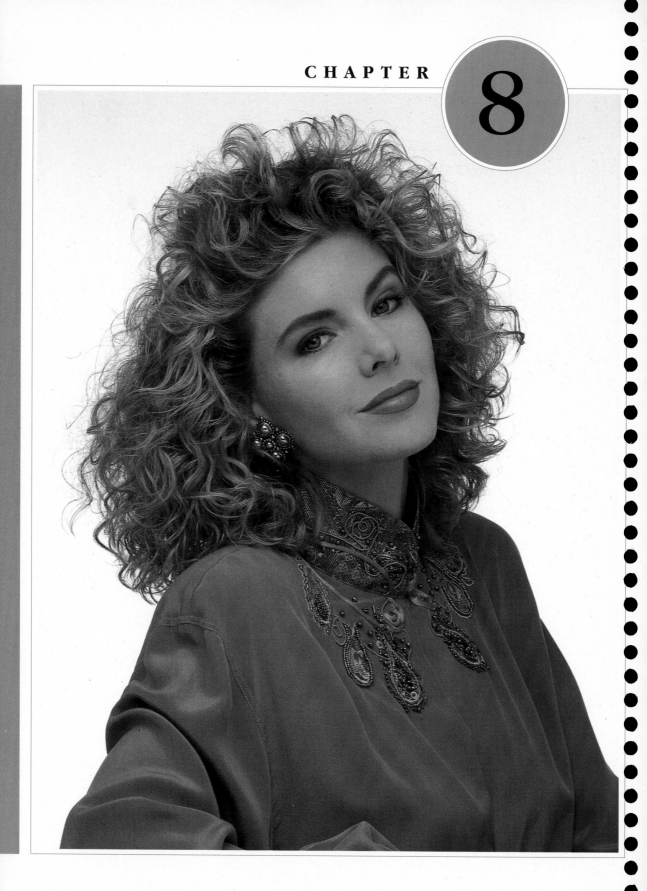

CHAPTER 8

A smart hair-care regimen, a great cut, and styling know-how are musts for achieving and maintaining healthy, good-looking hair. But coloring and perming techniques can transform hair from simply good-looking to gorgeous.

COLOR CUES

"Years ago, hair-coloring products were reserved for 'covering up the gray,' " notes Elsa Serra, Color Director for the Louis-Guy D Salon, in New York City. "But today, more and more women are scheduling color appointments when they call for a cut, *or* coloring their hair at home. They realize that artfully placed highlights or rich one-step color can warm their complexion, as well as add gloss, body, and depth to their hair," she explains.

Serra adds that the choices in hair color are myriad (see "Color Options," page 150). But whatever coloring process you choose—be it subtle highlights or an all-over tint—the more you know about salon or at-home coloring, the better your hair will look.

Start by getting your hair into the healthiest shape possible before coloring. If your hair is "virgin" (not color-treated, permed, or over-dried by chlorine from swimming pools, or the damaging rays from the sun), simply deep-condition three days prior to coloring. Choose an over-the-counter "deep-moisturizing" treatment, work evenly into hair from roots to ends, and leave in for 5 to 10 minutes. Use a protein-based conditioner after shampooing.

Eye-Catching Color, Head-Turning Curls

143

Processed or super-dry hair? Deep condition locks twice weekly for several weeks before coloring (use a "protein pack" or a remoisturizing treatment). Protein and remoisturizing products repair damaged hair, filling in the "cracks" or porous areas on too-dry hair, allowing it to color *evenly*.

Wash your hair a minimum of 24 hours before salon or at-home coloring (the natural oil that coats the hair during this time will help achieve better color penetration). Make sure your hair is free of heavy residue from conditioners, sprays, gels, and mousses. All can affect the way color takes.

Tell your colorist if you've used henna or any European botanical products (shampoos, conditioners, mousses) usually sold at health-food stores. Henna and certain botanicals can build up on the hair and interact with color to turn hair green.

First time for hair color? Schedule a skin patch test and a strand test several days before your appointment. A patch test can rule out skin sensitivity to the coloring product. A strand test will allow you to "preview" the results—and see if you like the way a particular color takes on your hair.

If you have a certain color in mind, or your colorist recommends one, ask to see her "swatch book," which will give you a fairly good idea of how the color will look.

Alert your colorist if you take certain medications that could affect your hair and alter the color. Some heart or chemotherapy drugs and blood-pressure medications can cause hair to take on unsightly tints (from yellow-green to bright red) during the coloring process. Iron supplements can interact with bleach or tints to produce a rusty-red residue on hair. Selenium supplements can trigger a turquoise cast. If you have *any* concerns as to how a particular medication will affect your hair color, a strand test is a *must*.

Ensure that your hair will retain its elasticity, look healthy and glossy, by having your colorist use a protein-based conditioner immediately after coloring (if you do at-home color, use a deep conditioning protein treatment, leaving product on hair for 5 to 10 minutes, depending on the dryness of your hair).

144

Whether you select highlights or all-over color (tints, semi-permanent color, etc.), for the most natural look, avoid going more than two or three shades lighter or darker than your own color. For example, if you have medium-brown hair, switch to a golden brown—but not to a dark blonde. If your hair is mousy brown, consider a warm brown shade with golden red highlights. For dark blondes, a move to medium blonde will light up your complexion, but a champagne color can look artificial and require too-frequent touch-ups—and may make you look washed out.

To keep color rich, prevent fading, use a shampoo and conditioner formulated for color-treated hair. Steer clear of dandruff shampoos containing sulfur, which can turn bleached or highlighted hair brassy, give brown-tinted hair a dull red cast. Instead, opt for dandruff products containing pyrithione zinc. (Note: Dandruff shampoos tend to be drying; if you use one every day, follow with a moisturizing conditioner.)

TURN UP THE LIGHTS!

Strategically placed highlights create a frame for the face, warming and brightening almost any complexion.

Highlights can be woven into the hair with the "foil" method (selected strands are placed on foil, color is applied, then hair is wrapped in foil), or simply painted onto the hair with a fine brush. Some salons use the old-fashioned "cap" method of highlighting (hairs are pulled through dozens of holes in a rubber or plastic cap, then lightened), but according to Elsa Serra, "Caps tend to produce heavy highlights in the crown area, rather than around the face. Look for a salon that uses the foil method for more precise and natural-looking highlights."

Here, highlighting how-to's:

· Highlights add body and volume to the hair both visually and physiologically. The coloring process "roughs up" the hair shaft, making it feel thicker. The interplay of darker and lighter hair creates the illusion of fullness. Use "whole head" highlights (see page 154) to plump up fine, thin hair.

· Having highlights done for the first time? Opt for a subtle look. Ask for very fine highlights around the face only (to brighten your complexion), or a "half head" (color is applied to front, sides, and crown area, blending naturally with back hair).

· Avoid too-pale or "white" highlights; they'll wash you out, and leave skin dull, unhealthy-looking.

· If your hair is medium to dark blonde and your complexion's on the cool side (with a pinky-blue undertone), choose ashy highlights (ashy colors are devoid of red). Warm skin with a golden undertone? Opt for highlights that are warm, intense.

· Don't be tempted to "go blonde" if you have brown hair. Golden (or white) streaks can look artificial in brunette hair, make skin appear pasty. Instead, choose a rich interplay of red-brown and gold-brown highlights.

· Stay away from all-one-color highlights. They can look fake. Beautiful mixes of two to four colors give hair depth, movement, and drama.

· To minimize frequent root touchups, ask for fine—rather than chunky—highlights. They'll grow out almost imperceptibly, roots won't be noticeable.

CAMOUFLAGING THE GRAY

Your natural hair color, plus the percentage of gray, will determine the type of coloring product you should use:

Blonde hair that's 25 to 50 percent gray? Opt for highlights. They'll blend with the gray for a natural

All-Over Color

One-step coloring processes (from temporary rinses to permanent dyes or tints) have been so refined in the past decade, women can now choose products that add a little color, a lot of color—or merely provide a hint of color plus lots of body and volume.

Use one-step color (home or salon) to give fine, limp hair body, add highlights, or cover gray.

146

look. Blonde hair that's 50 percent gray? A few lucky blondes can highlight their hair well into their fifties or sixties. Others can achieve beautiful blonde locks with a combination of strategically placed highlights and a semi-permanent rinse for a more blended look.

If your hair is *light brown* and 25 to 50 percent gray, select a dark golden blonde or golden brown semi-permanent all-over rinse to knock out some of the gray and create highlights.

For *medium brown hair* that's 25 to 30 percent gray, consider using a semi-permanent all-over color to lighten hair by one or two shades (choose salon or home products in auburn or light golden brown). The lighter color will flatter your complexion. Once a woman passes forty, her skin tends to lose color, and darker hair can make her look tired and pale.

Dark brown hair that's 25 to 30 percent gray? You'll need semi-permanent all-over color, or highlights *plus* a semi-permanent rinse to camouflage the gray.

Medium to dark brown hair that's 40 percent plus gray? A permanent tint will give you the greatest coverage.

Like your gray hair, but want just a little more pizazz? See "Gray Optimizers" on page 152.

COLORING ASIAN HAIR

Asian hair grays slowly, so you probably won't need all-over color until your fifties or sixties. Never use *black* rinses or tints; your hair will look dull, opaque. Instead, select the darkest brown shade available, if you have black hair. For medium brown hair, choose a shade that's close to your natural color; avoid products with too much red pigment.

Want to add highlights? Consider a minimum of subtle, blue-based burgundy lights here and there.

Whatever your color choice, keep in mind that Asian hair has a "tighter" hair cuticle and therefore it is harder for color to penetrate—best to put your hair in the hands of a coloring pro.

AFRICAN-AMERICAN HAIR:
COLOR WITH CARE

"Black hair is extremely fragile," notes Serra. "It's akin to *sensitive skin* and needs to be handled with utmost care."

· Choose a salon that specializes in coloring black hair.

· Have your hair color done by a professional—at least the first time; ask your colorist to recommend a coloring product you can safely use at home.

· Black hair loses color easily. Opt for products and processes using a *minimum* of peroxide. Too-strong products can promote drastic color change, trigger breakage.

· Stay close to your own color for a natural look, minimal damage to hair. If your hair is light brown—and in very good condition—you can switch to a dark-dark blonde color with a minimum of wear and tear on your hair. If your hair is very dark and you'd like to cover the gray, opt for a semi-permanent color *(permanent tints are too drying for black hair)*.

· Prefer highlights? Ask your colorist to use a low-volume peroxide product to give you reddish-brown tones.

· Don't use henna on black hair. It can leave hair straw-like.

· If you plan to color chemically straightened hair, deep condition it twice weekly for several weeks prior to coloring. Straighten hair a minimum of two weeks before having it colored. (If you color too soon after straightening, your hair will take the color too quickly, may look overly dark.) *Never* straighten hair immediately after coloring; the chemicals in the straightener will "pull" color from your hair, leaving it faded. (Note: If you straighten your hair, be sure to tell your colorist.)

PERFECT COLOR—AT HOME

Many hair coloring processes can be done at home—at a substantial savings when compared to salon costs. But whether you choose a temporary rinse, highlighting, or semi-permanent or permanent color, check our these home hair coloring tips for salon results:

If you plan to make a "color jump"—going three shades lighter or darker than your natural hair color—or you've never colored your hair before, put yourself in the hands of a professional colorist the first time around. The colorist can then recommend salon or over-the-counter products you can use to duplicate the results at home.

When buying a color kit, be sure you choose the correct shade. Look for your *natural* color on the box chart, then check to see how that particular product color will alter it. (Don't be fooled by the photo on the front of the box.)

Choose a shade that complements your skin tone. If your complexion is cool (with a pinky-blue undertone), opt for ashy shades that are devoid of red. If you have warm skin with a golden undertone, choose warm colors with hints of gold, auburn, or red.

When covering gray, pick a color that adds depth and richness, rather than simply matching your hair color exactly. For example, if your hair's mousy brown, and you use an ash-brown hair color, you *could* end up with a flat cast or greenish tinge. The ashy color will have destroyed the hair's ability to catch, reflect light. A better option? A light brown tint with a golden or reddish hue.

Do a strand test before applying color to see whether you like the results.

Do a patch test 24 hours prior to using any coloring product to rule out skin sensitivity. Apply a dab to the inside of your arm (near the elbow). If redness,

Eye-Catching Color, Head-Turning Curls

itching, swelling, or irritation results, don't use the product.

Follow instructions to the letter. If the instructions say "Leave on for 10 minutes," don't wash the color out 5 minutes early, hoping to get a lighter shade.

Pay special attention to any caution notices. For example, since semi-permanent hair color can react adversely with permanent tints, avoid using one product over the other.

Have all coloring supplies handy before you begin. Gather towels, bowls, timer, comb, etc., so you'll avoid having to search for something (and risk dripping your way through the house).

If you're doing home highlights, use highlighter sparingly, applying fine lights around the face (pay special attention to bangs and hairline). Later, if you'd like more highlights, apply them where needed.

When buying any type of hair-color kit, check the package expiration date. "Old" color won't give the best results.

Color Options

Temporary Colors. Use these rinses, mousses, sprays, paint-on brighteners, and gels to add depth and richness to your natural color, or for highlighting purposes. All coat the cuticle of the hair, make it temporarily "thicker," so they add body to fine locks. Some contain conditioners that add gloss as well. Temporaries won't provide enough coverage to conceal gray and they can't lighten hair. They wash out with your next shampoo and can be done at salons or at home.

Vegetable Glazes or Dyes. A good bet for a subtle color change, these semi-permanent colors last from two to six weeks, give hair shine and body. The color is brushed onto wet hair, then heat-activated (clients sit under a dryer) for 30 to 60 minutes. Gentle enough to be used on permed or highlighted hair (to perk up fading lights), vegetable glazes can also darken hair by one or two shades and wash away gradually. Can be done at salons only.

Semi-permanent Colors. Containing little or no peroxide, these products can't lighten hair, but will

150

deepen, darken, or enrich your natural color while adding body. Some contain conditioners that give hair shine, and a few newer products provide gloss and volume with little or no color. By using a color one shade lighter than your natural hair hue, you can achieve subtle gold or reddish highlights. Semi-permanents can cover up to 50 percent of gray, depending on your natural hair color, and they can last four to six weeks. Can be done at salons or at home.

One-Step Permanent Colors. Because these colors contain peroxide, they penetrate to the cortex, or center, of the hair and can be used to darken *or* lighten hair. Permanent colors cover gray completely, give dark hair depth and intensity, warm up light brown and blonde locks. (Some products contain gloss-boosting conditioners.) The color stays true—it won't wash away—but roots may need touch-ups every four weeks or so, depending on your hair growth and color. Can be done at salons or at home.

Double-Process Blonding. The hair is bleached or partially lightened to strip away the natural color, then tinted to bring hair to a pale, delicate blonde. This

151

process can take dark brown hair to champagne blonde and is a dramatic color change. Best for strong, healthy hair that can stand up to intensive bleaching. The color is permanent, and roots will have to be retouched as needed. Best done at salons (the overlap of color could result in excessive breakage).

Henna. Hair color made from the leaves and stems of the henna plant, these products give hair a reddish tint—from pale strawberry (on natural blondes) to an intense red-black (on darker hair). Henna penetrates the hair shaft and can't be washed away (even colorless henna—used to boost body—is permanent). Henna *can* add shine and body to hair, but it also coats the hair, causing a color buildup after repeated treatments. A henna coating on the hair can interfere with other coloring processes, as well as perming, and used too often it can leave hair dry and brittle. Can be done at salons or at home.

Gray Optimizers. Semi-permanent color that minimizes yellowish tones in gray hair (can be used on hair that's predominantly gray, or partially gray). The color makes gray hair appear silvery and glossy, so it catches and reflects light better (naturally gray hair can become a little dry and dull). You won't need touchups to conceal roots, but you will need to recolor as needed to maintain the effect. Can be done at salons and at home.

Highlighting. This process is also called "streaking" or "frosting" (a thicker, "stripier," contrast of color), "tipping" (on short hair or ends of hair), and "hairpainting" (a freestyle method).

At salons, strands are pulled from hair with a rat-tail comb, painted with lightener or color, then wrapped in foil (some salons use the old-fashioned cap method of highlighting, while others prefer hairpainting—brushing color onto sections of hair, without the use of a cap or foil).

Home highlighting kits include a cap with tiny holes plus a crochet-hook-like instrument, which you use to pull hair through holes. Hairpainting kits include a fine-tipped brush.

There are various types of highlighting methods (and many salons have different names for them), and the one you choose should be determined by your

152

hair color, how subtle or dramatic you prefer the highlights to be, and how often you're able to have touch-ups:

Color wrapping: Perhaps the most natural highlighting process, since two to four tints, similar to your own color, are woven through the hair to create a subtle, but rich, interplay of colors. Works well on dark blondes and women with light brown locks. Highlights grow out gradually and touchups are recommended as needed. Some at-home "low-lights" kits can approximate salon color wrapping, but for best results, have a professional do the job.

Tortoise-shelling: Essentially color-wrapping for darker hair. Fine streaks of deep reds, golds, and brandy shades are woven through medium or dark brown hair to create depth and movement. Touch up new growth every three to six months or as needed. Should be done at a salon by an expert colorist for best results.

Thermal color: One of the newest highlighting techniques, this process mimics color wrapping and tortoise-shelling, but there's less potential for damage to the hair, since the coloring product contains very little peroxide. The color—from golden blonde to warm brown—is painted onto selected strands of hair, then wrapped in foil. The client sits under a dryer for 20 to 30 minutes (the heat, rather than peroxide, opens the cuticle, allowing the color to penetrate deeply). Thermal color is gentle enough to use on bleached or highlighted hair to add warmth, depth, and shine. It can also create highlights in hair that's been permanently colored (with a one-step process), but has started to look dull. Touch up every three to four months. Available at some salons.

Sunbursting: Minimal, super-fine highlights are randomly placed throughout hair to achieve a sun-kissed look. Works well on dark blonde, light brown, and even medium brown hair, adding just a *hint* of gold. Grows out gradually, so no touch-ups are required. Best for women who want a sun-streaked look—without exposing their hair to the sun's damaging rays. Can be done at a salon or at home with a hair-painting kit—a nice pick-up during the winter months.

153

Hairpainting (or balayaging): Similar to sun-bursting, but less bright and usually done on very light hair. Highlights are painted, with a fine brush, on top of head only. Looks best on short or medium-length hair (for longer hair, opt for sunbursting). Touch up every three to five months. Best done at salons, though you *can* create similar streaks with a hairpainting kit—and a very light touch.

Whole-head highlighting: Highlights are placed throughout entire head, so this is the most extensive, time-consuming, and expensive form of highlighting. This process works well for women with layered styles, where underneath hair is visible, and those with fine, limp hair that needs a "body boost" provided by color. Touch-ups are frequent—every four to twelve weeks, depending on how dark your roots are. (You *can* opt for a "hairline" touch-up between color treatments; see below.) Can be done at salons or at home.

Half-head highlighting: Streaks are placed at the sides and crown and in bang area. Best for one-length styles, since highlighted hair must blend with back hair for a natural look. Touch-ups can be done every six to twelve weeks, depending on the amount and thickness of the highlights (you can conceal roots with a "hairline," done midway between color treatments). Best done at salons, though you can use a home high-lighting kit (be sure to have a friend help you, so highlights extend far enough into the crown to blend with back hair).

Hairline highlighting: A touch-up process, highlights are painted onto the part, into bangs, and around the face, camouflaging *most* visible roots until next major highlighting is done.

SMART CURES FOR COLOR CATASTROPHES

Problem: Hair that's over-bleached or over-high-lighted.

Solution: Bring hair closer to its natural color with *lowlights,* darker strands woven throughout hair. (Lowlights kits are available at drugstores, but a profes-sional colorist can achieve the most natural look.)

Problem: You used a semi-permanent rinse and hate the shade. While the color *will* fade in six to eight weeks, you'd like to go back to your natural color—now!

Solution: Use a hair-color remover kit (available at drugstores), or better yet, have a professional colorist remove the color. Then, select a semi-permanent rinse close to your natural shade and recolor your hair.

Problem: You used a spray-on hair lightener—the type that brightens hair while you sit in the sun—and now, summer's over and your roots are showing. You can't afford salon highlights right now, but you do want to keep your hair slightly blonde, allowing it to "grow out" naturally.

Solution: Use a hairpainting kit to place subtle highlights randomly along your part, in bangs, and at temples. The highlights will blend with the blonder hair. Repeat every six to eight weeks.

Problem: You have your gray hair colored professionally with a semi-permanent or permanent color. Your roots are showing, but you can't book an appointment with your colorist.

Solution: Buy a color touch-up crayon (also called a color touch-up stick), available at many drugstores, in your exact shade. Gently color visible gray (color will last until you wash it out).

Problem: Your highlighted hair begins to look brassy (because of too much time spent in the sun, exposure to chlorine, etc.).

Solution: Use a color-corrective shampoo, formulated to tone down yellow or brassiness in either gray or highlighted hair (look for one with a violet/blue hue). Is hair just this side of orange? Ask your colorist to take out the brass with a semi-permanent color rinse in a slightly ashy shade.

Problem: You had your hair highlighted (at a salon or home), and the streaks are too white, leaving you with a pale, unhealthy look.

Solution: Have a professional colorist weave lowlights (see above) throughout your hair, or use a temporary or semi-permanent color in a gold shade to add warmth.

Problem: The highlights that looked so shiny and warm just two months ago are drab, faded.

Solution: Revive tired highlights with a vegetable glaze (golden blonde for blonde hair, auburn for reddish-brown locks). Vegetable glazing is available at salons.

MAKING WAVES

Not so long ago, a permanent wave was synonymous with crisp, unyielding curls. But today, with the new, technologically advanced perms available, you can have curls and waves so natural-looking, people will swear you were born with them.

Milder perming solutions ensure that nineties perms are far less damaging to the hair than the older versions. Variations in wrapping techniques offer dozens of options in the amount and type of curl achieved (for example, hair that's twirled, then wrapped around a small rod, will yield *corkscrew* curls). What's more, the newest perms incorporate conditioners and proteins that maximize your hair's health.

A good perm can add texture and body to fine, droopy hair, give direction to straight coarse tresses, and transform frizzy hair into soft waves. Here, a guide to salon and home perms.

A PERMING PRIMER

Conventional "Cold" Waves produce a well-defined curl that *lasts*. Some stronger formulations work well on limp, hard-to-curl hair; milder solutions can be used on color-treated locks. Many of the home cold-wave kits have automatic curl "timers" that stop the curling process once the right amount of wave is achieved. Available at salons and in at-home kits.

Acid-Balanced Perms are milder and gentler than the cold-wave variety and work well on fine, medium-textured, tinted, or dry hair (in certain cases,

> *No matter what your choice in color, be prepared to take a close look at your skin tone and make some changes in your color cosmetics. Going lighter often calls for softer, clearer tones of blush or lipstick. Darker, shiny hair can mean brighter, deeper shades.*

156

acid perms can be used on highlighted hair that's in *exceptionally* good health). This heat-activated process yields soft, loose waves—and there's less likelihood of frizzing. Available at salons.

Exothermic Perms are the strongest formulation—an alkaline wave formula mixed with a chemical heat component. This type of perm creates well-defined, springy curls and should be used only on healthy, coarse, hard-to-curl hair. Available at some salons.

Soft Waves or bisulfite perms are a mainstay of many home perming products. Very mild, these perms are less likely than cold waves to cause breakage or frizzing and are ideal for fragile, sun-damaged, or color-treated hair. Soft waves tend to last only two or three months. (If not properly done, they can fizzle after a couple of weeks!)

How well a perm takes depends, in part, on the skill of the stylist. Choose a salon with a perming staff, or at least one person who specializes in perms.

THE WRAP

Be sure to choose the right rod for the amount (or type) of curl you want to achieve. Most stylists use traditional perming rods, but some innovators wrap hair around everything from special zig-zag rods (they look like lightning streaks!) to thick popsicle sticks. Here, the results of more conventional wraps:

· Straight rods produce evenly formed curls.

· Concave rods create curls that are straighter at the roots, wavier at the ends.

· Narrow rods yield tight curls.

· Medium-width rods, medium or loose curls.

· Large rods produce soft waves.

· Pincurl perms (in which sections of hair are wrapped around a finger, then secured with a hairpin or clip) offer very soft, loose waves.

MORE PERM CHOICES

Curly perms give you wash 'n' wear hair. With an expert cut, all you need do is shampoo, condition, detangle, "set" with a little mousse or spray gel, and air dry. (Or, you can use a brush and blow-dryer to achieve controlled waves.) Note: Avoid short layers that are all one length; you can end up looking like a poodle! A better bet: longer, graduated layers. Curly perms can be done at salons and at home.

Body waves add curves and volume and are a good choice for giving lift to fine, droopy hair. Available at salons, in home perm kits.

Root perms are done on "root hair" only, giving lift and volume without curls or waves. Ideal for straight hair that tends to lie flat, lack body. (Root perms are also a quick fix for curly perms or body waves that are growing out.) Don't attempt a root perm at home—this one needs professional know-how.

Underneath perms give fullness and body to blunt, one-length cuts that need support from beneath. The lower layers of hair are loosely permed, so this is a good choice for women who have highlighted the top layer of their hair—and don't want to risk perming the bleached areas. You can do an underneath perm at home, using a body wave and perming the hair below the ears only. Get a friend to help section hair evenly. Also available at salons.

Flat-wrap perms mimic naturally wavy hair with soft, loose curls. But instead of wrapping the hair away from the face (the case with most perms), the hair is wrapped toward the face to give a strong wave—and lift—at the hairline. Can be done at home or at salons.

Weave perms wave only portions of the hair to give natural fullness and curves, rather than precise curls. Weave perms can be tricky, so put your hair in the hands of an expert.

Reverse perms will relax tight natural curls, and can be done on any length of hair that hasn't been chemically relaxed or straightened. The hair is wrapped around big rods, then permed to make curls looser, softer.

Directional perms are problem-solvers, helping hair that usually falls in your eyes to curve gracefully away from your face, or locks that flip up to turn neatly under. For best results, have a perming pro do the job.

Spot perms provide lift or curl at particular points only, and are ideal for giving body and direction to droopy bangs, height at the crown, or volume in the temple area. Spot perms can be done at salons or at home.

ASIAN HAIR—CURL CAREFULLY

"Many Western stylists mistakenly assume that because Asian hair is often coarse it *resists* curling—so they use perms for hard-to-curl hair, or leave the perming solution on too long," says Yosh, owner of the Yosh For Hair salons in San Francisco and Palo Alto, California.

Both invite disaster, he observes. "Some Asian hair can take a curl *very* quickly and calls for mild acid-balanced salon perms or very gentle at-home formulas." Be sure to check curls periodically to see how fast the perm is taking, he adds. "A few minutes can mean the difference between wavy, softly curled hair—and a mass of frizz."

THE NEW WAVE IN PERMS

Milder solutions, in both salon and home perms, ensure that permed hair stays healthy. New perms incorporate conditioners that leave hair softer, glossier, and more manageable. Many perms contain proteins that fill in damaged or porous areas on the hair shaft, making it stronger and more able to withstand perming (these perms are good options for women with color-treated or dry hair). What to look for in the future? Perms containing herbal extracts and vitamins that will give hair more shine. Also on the horizon: chemical-free organic perms made from vegetable, plant, and mineral proteins.

AT-HOME PERM—SALON RESULTS

Home perms are similar to the ones used in salons, though the solutions are milder. Follow these easy tips to achieve a salon-quality perm at home:

· Ask a friend to section and roll your hair (especially the back areas).

· Use two end papers per roller, one on top of hair, one underneath, to curb frizzing. Super-short hair? Wrap entire length of hair in end paper.

· Thoroughly saturate wrapped hair with solution; otherwise, you'll end up with unevenly waved locks. Instead of wrapping hair around the rod the way you'd wrap hair around a roller, wrap it in a spiral, starting at one end of the rod and finishing at the other. The perming solution will penetrate this type of wrap much more easily.

· Roll rods in the direction you want your hair to go. Roll hair forward for tousled styles that frame the face; away from the face for a brushed-back look.

· Keep solution off your face and scalp (it can cause irritation). Each time you apply solution, use a damp washcloth or big wet cotton balls to wipe solution off scalp (and to blot up any drips that trickle onto your face).

· Color-treated tresses? Color-treated hair is porous and takes a curl quickly, so you'll want to leave the perming solution on for a shorter time than indicated in the instructions—better yet, leave your perm to the pros.

· Most home-perm kits have built-in "curl shut-offs." That is, once a curl forms, the solution stops working. But to be on the safe side, unwrap several curls three-quarters of the way through the perming process to make sure the perm isn't taking too quickly.

160

· Avoid leaving neutralizer on the hair too long. It can over-process the perm and damage your hair.

· Follow all directions *exactly*. Home perms are carefully tested and directions must be followed to achieve the best results.

TO RE-PERM OR NOT TO RE-PERM?

Avoid having an all-over perm more than three times a year, depending on the condition of the hair, say the pros. Perming too often can result in damaged hair that's dry, brittle, broken.

· *Cold Wave Perms*—use once or twice a year max (once is preferable, according to many hair experts).
· *Acid-Balanced Perms*—use two or three times a year.
· *Soft Wave or Bisulfite Perms*—you'll need to reperm three or four times yearly, since this wave wilts after a few months.

Have hair trimmed every four to six weeks; excess length can weigh down curls. Frequent cuts will help keep curls springy.

T.L.C. FOR CURLY TOPS

1. To prevent breakage and frizzing, your hair must be in excellent condition before perming. Strengthen with weekly moisturizing treatments.
2. Don't perm bleached or highlighted hair—unless it's *exceptionally* strong and healthy. (Test strength by snipping a single hair, then pulling on it at both ends. If it snaps, perming chemicals will cause breakage.)
3. Allow the perm to "settle in" for the first day or two (no blow-drying, shampooing, if possible) in order for the curl to last.
4. Be sure to have a post-perm trim to snip away any frizzy ends.

161

5. Use shampoos formulated for permed hair (these products preserve the curl) or a gentle shampoo.

6. Use a detangling rinse or light protein conditioner after *every* shampoo to prevent tangling, matting.

7. Blot shampooed hair with a fluffy towel—never *rub* permed hair; it'll tangle.

8. Curly hair doesn't catch and reflect light the way straight hair does. Give your permed locks shine by working a dab of gel or "laminate" through dry hair. (This can curb frizzies in humid weather.)

9. To add more body to *fine* permed hair, work mousse or gel through damp hair, using your fingers to shape curls, give hair direction, give the perm control. Air dry.

CROSS-COUNTRY BEAUTY

Color-treated hair is porous and soaks up moisture from the air. If you live in a close-to-tropical region, such as *Florida* or *Louisiana*, to keep fine, straight hair from wilting, curly hair from frizzing, try using a *lighter* lotion conditioner after shampooing. Protein-based conditioners fill in the porous areas on the hair shaft, helps "seal out" humidity.

Hair that's body-waved can sag in cold, super-dry weather. If you're from the *Midwest*, use a perm-reviving lotion or spritz to keep waves wavy, curls bouncy, *or* be sure to lock H_2O into hair with a "remoisturizing conditioner."

Live in *Southern California*? Rehydrate sun-parched permed or color-treated hair by mixing a dab of alcohol-free gel with a "dime's worth" of aloe vera gel (available in 99 percent strength at drugstores). Work through hair for direction, hold—and gloss.

BEAUTY WRAP-UP

1. Coloring products don't just cover gray—they also add body, shine, to hair. Use conditioning colors to give curly hair gloss, highlights, and one-step color

Real Beauty . . . Real Women

to boost body in fine, limp locks.

2. For the most natural look, avoid going more than two shades darker or lighter than your natural color.

3. Strategically placed highlights can warm, brighten almost any complexion.

4. Use highlights or all-over color to restore richness to winter-drab hair.

5. African-American hair that's chemically straightened must be colored with utmost care. Always straighten hair first, wait two weeks, then color. The chemicals in straighteners can "lift" color from your hair.

6. Avoid one-color or too-white highlights. They'll make you look washed out. Instead, opt for dramatic interplays of two to four rich colors.

7. If you have hard-to-curl hair, or want a springy wave, choose a cold wave.

8. If your hair is dry, color-treated, or fragile, choose mild acid-balanced salon perms or bisulfite home perming kits (soft waves).

9. Keep all-over perming to a minimum for the sake of your hair's health. In between perms, revive droopy curls with spot or root perms, and by having ends trimmed regularly.

10. Curly hair doesn't reflect light the way straight locks do, so you'll need to work with gels or laminates to restore shine and elasticity.

11. Be sure you alert your hairstylist if you take medications. Some (not all) can affect your hair and alter the outcome of a perm or the color.

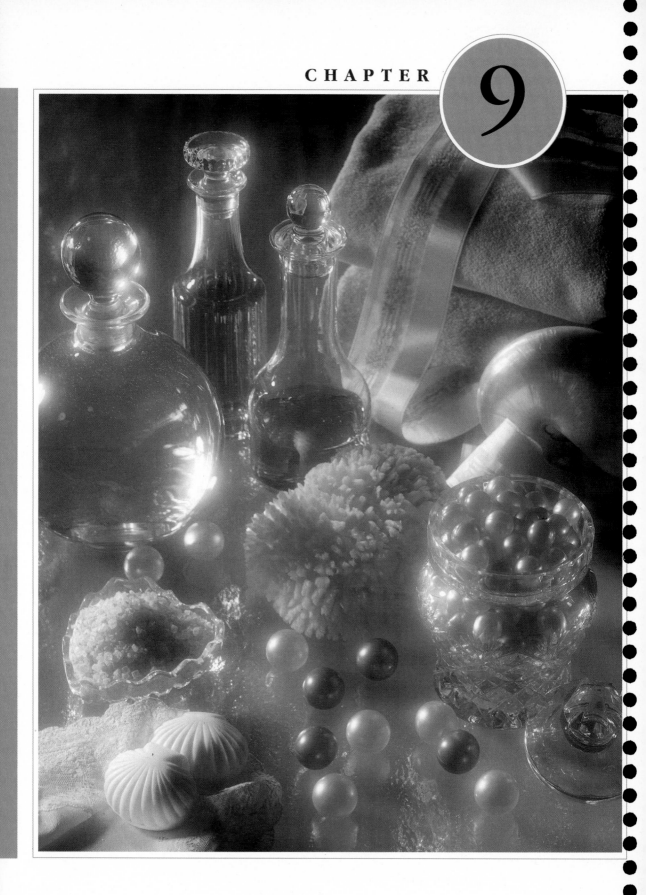

CHAPTER 9

Your complexion is radiant. Your hair looks terrific. Your makeup is flawless. But wait—what about the *rest* of your body, your shoulders, back, legs, hands, and feet? It's easy to forget (and neglect) these areas. After all, when we look at ourselves in the mirror, it's usually from the neck up. But a smart beauty regimen focuses on the total package, giving just as much care and attention to body skin, hands, feet—*and* nails. Here, a guide that will "do a body good."

SHOWER POWER

Your morning shower wakes you up, gets you going.

- Opt for a quick shower and keep water comfortably warm, not hot—hot water will dehydrate your skin.

- Choose a soap or cleanser formulated for your body's skin type. Use a moisturizing soap, beauty bar, or hydrating gel for dry or mature skin, a gentle glycerin or oil-balancing soap or soapless gel for skin that tends to get oily on the chest and back.

Body Beautiful

- Rough patches on thighs, buttocks, elbows, and knees? Use cleansing grains incorporated into a creamy base to slough away dry skin (look for "scrubs" that come in tubes instead of jars—you can get a better grip on tube containers when showering). Or, opt for a loofah sponge to *gently* remove scaly skin.

- Rub a pumice stone over roughened heels and on calluses on balls of feet.

- Rinse your body well, pat (don't rub) away excess moisture, then smooth body lotion over still-damp skin. Do you like the softening effects of bath oil? Use an after-shower bath oil *spray* and mist over damp skin to lock in water.

THE ARTFUL BATH

Even if you're a confirmed shower person, treat yourself to a leisurely bath at least once a week—to renew body and mind.

Gather a "bath pillow" or large rolled towel to cushion your head and neck; bath oil; a loofah or bath sponge; and a pumice stone. (If you like to read while bathing, buy a plastic bath tray to hold your favorite book or magazine.)

Light scented candles for a tranquil atmosphere, and tune your radio to a station that plays relaxing, commercial-free music.

Cleanse your face as usual and smooth on a mask suited to your skin type.

Draw a warm—not hot—bath (the ideal temperature is 95 to 100 degrees). As the tub fills, pour a capful of bath oil into water to soothe and moisturize dry skin. Or add six to eight drops of any essential oil (rose, jasmine, lavender) to bath water to create your own spa-like "aromatherapy."

Lie back and soak for 10 to 15 minutes. Don't extend your bath past 20 minutes—your skin will pucker up like a prune.

Fast Fixes in the Bath

· Using a pumice stone, smooth rough heels and sides of feet.

· Use a loofah or cleansing grains to slough away dry skin on thighs, elbows, and knees.

· Now's the time to pluck stray brow hairs (the warmth and moisture from your bath will soften hairs, make them easier to tweeze). Use a magnifying mirror and slant-edged tweezers.

· Missed exercise class? Try these easy tub exercises.

Shower Therapy

Need to unkink taut muscles? Treat yourself to a special shower attachment that massages you as you shower. Set your shower attachment on "pulsating" and aim the water at the muscles between your shoulders for about 20 seconds, each side. Aim a strong spray of water at your upper back and the base of your neck (bend head slightly forward) for approximately 20 seconds. The pressure and warmth of the water will soothe tired muscles and help ease any pain or tenderness due to exercising.

166

—Abdomen Tightener. Brace head against plastic bath pillow or rolled towel. Hold sides of tub and raise legs. Bend left knee, then straighten. Repeat with right leg. Do three times.

—Thigh Firmer. While sitting, raise one leg, grab calf, and pull leg slowly toward you. Do three times with each leg.

APRÈS BATH

·Use a big, fluffy towel to pat away excess moisture, then slather on body lotion or cream, paying special attention to elbows, knees, hands, and heels of feet.

·Ease slowly into your daily routine by wrapping yourself in a thick terry robe, brewing a cup of herbal tea, and cuddling up on the sofa with that new novel or magazine you've been anxious to read.

SPA BATH

Tired, sore muscles? Rough, dry skin? Treat yourself to this kind-to-skin-and-muscles bath, suggested by skin pro Ole Henriksen: Run a comfortably warm bath, mixing 1 pound* of Epsom salts and 1 ounce of either pure rosemary or eucalyptus oil into water. Turn on shower and thoroughly wet your skin; then, gently rub sea salt (available at health-food stores) over chest, shoulders, back, thighs, and legs; use a firm circular motion (expect a slight tingling sensation). Lower yourself into bath and relax for 10 to 15 minutes. Sea salt softens skin and exfoliates dry flakes. Epsom salts soothe achy muscles. Eucalyptus is a natural astringent, and rosemary cleanses and conditions skin.

CALMING MILK BATH

"Add 2 cups instant dry milk to comfortably warm

*Sounds like a lot—it isn't.

bath water to smooth and soothe skin. Cut two pieces of cheesecloth (about 5" by 5" square) and fill with 1/4 to 1/2 cup bran; use string to tie the double-layered bag securely shut. Allow the sachet to float in tub while you relax for 15 minutes. Then, rub sachet over your body to smooth dry patches. (You can add several drops of lavender or rose oil to bath water for a *scent*sational experience.)"

—*Ole Henriksen*

SUNBURN SOOTHER

Too much time in the sun? Take the sting and redness out of a very mild burn with this healing bath: Pour 1 quart whole milk into a tub filled with cool to tepid water. Add 1/2 cup aloe vera gel (use your hand to distribute gel throughout the bath). Opt for a mild oatmeal soap to gently cleanse skin. (Oatmeal helps calm irritated complexions.) Relax for 10 minutes.

COLD-WEATHER SKIN CARE

· In addition to applying moisturizer to damp skin right after your morning shower, help prevent a winter-dry body by reapplying lotion or cream at night.

· Use extra-rich moisture creams on knees, elbows, and heels.

· Be sure to exfoliate legs every few days to remove dry skin buildup; use cleansing grains in a moisturizing base, or a loofah. Extra-sensitive skin? Opt for a bath sponge rather than a loofah.

· Keep the chill out by wearing several layers of clothing. If you begin to feel warm, remove layers—that way, you'll prevent excessive sweating, which can irritate your skin, cause breakouts on your back, shoulders, and chest.

· Keep humidifiers going in the bedroom and living room to add moisture to your environment.

·Set the thermostat at 68 degrees. Higher temperatures will rob your skin of moisture and leave it flaky, dull, with a "tight" feeling.

·Avoid too-frequent baths or showers, which can make your skin look like the Mohave Desert.

WARM-WEATHER SKIN SAVERS

·Keep a jar of pre-moistened astringent pads at your office. After running lunch-time errands, slip into the restroom and whisk a pad over your chest, back, and neck to remove oil and perspiration. You'll feel cool instantly.

·Refrigerate toner or astringent. After a hectic day, saturate a big cosmetics puff with cool astringent and smooth over face, chest, back, and neck.

·Air-conditioners take a toll on skin by sapping moisture from the air. Use humidifiers to boost the moisture level in your home.

·To feel fresh and perspiration-free on warm, humid days, dust inner thighs, under breast area, and underarms with your favorite fragrant talc or cornstarch baby powder.

·Choose a *combination* antiperspirant/deodorant to keep underarms odor and perspiration free. Always apply to *dry* skin (water will dilute the moisture-blocking ingredients in antiperspirants). Be sure to use every day: it takes up to one week of daily use for the antiperspirant ingredients to become totally effective.

In general, solid "stick" products are more effective than aerosols. Roll-ons offer the best protection of all, but be sure to shake a roll-on before using it. The antiperspirant ingredients tend to settle at the bottom of the container.

Keep a clean, fluffy towel handy when exercising, and frequently pat away perspiration (the salts in sweat can irritate your skin). Try to shower immediately following workouts to wash away oil and sweat, which can combine to clog pores, trigger breakouts on your back and chest.

169

Prone to breakouts on your back? Use an oil-balancing soap or cleanser and be sure to wash all areas of your back (use a big, easy-to-grip sponge or a long-handled soft-bristled bath brush). Before bedtime, smooth benzoyl peroxide cream or lotion over clean, dry skin (allow benzoyl peroxide to dry completely before donning nightclothes—it can bleach clothing).

Once a week, treat your back to a pore-cleansing mask. Shower, pat skin dry, then smooth on a clay-based mask, one that contains salicylic acid, or the easy-to-make "back mask" below. Leave on for 5 to 10 minutes (you can use this time to start your weekly pedicure)—then rinse skin thoroughly.

Back Smoother

Mix together: 1/2 cup powdered dry milk, 1 beaten egg white, and 1 ounce witch hazel (or mild astringent).

In the shower, use a loofah to slough away dry skin. Smooth mask over skin and allow to dry. Rinse thoroughly.

TAKE IT OFF!
(GETTING RID OF BODY HAIR)

There are a number of ways to remove (or camouflage) unwanted hair, and the method you choose will depend on how much time (and money) you want to spend. For a description of some of the most common hair-removal techniques—bleaching, tweezing, depilatories, waxing, and electrolysis—see "De-Fuzzing," page 48. Then check out our body-smoothing suggestions, below.

Light to medium-brown hair on forearms? Consider bleaching with an at-home kit (choose a product formulated for use on the *body*). Bleach *can* turn *dark* brown hair orange, and repeated treatments may be necessary to achieve a natural-looking color. Depilatories and waxes can also be used to remove forearm hair and are a better choice if your hair is very dark. Bleach, waxes, and depilatories can irritate sensitive or mature skin, so do a patch test before using.

Need to clean up your bikini line? Salon or home waxing leaves skin ultra-smooth, hair-free for several weeks. Depilatories formulated for the bikini area also work well. But both waxing and depilatories can irritate sensitive bikini-area skin. Be careful *not* to apply too close to the vaginal area, and do a skin test before using either product. (Be extra careful if you decide to shave the bikini area. Many skin experts advise *against* shaving this area. Shaving can leave the skin itchy and irritated—and a stubbly regrowth usually appears within a day or two.)

Avoid sun exposure or swimming in chlorinated pools for 24 hours after using wax or a depilatory in the bikini area.

Want to remove underarm hair? Some women prefer depilatories because they leave underarms ultra-smooth, but these products may cause irritation. Shaving is a better bet (see "Close Shaves," page 171).

Fuzz on knuckles of fingers or toes? Depilatories are a good choice for removing knuckle hair. Electrolysis, though costly and time-consuming, can be used to permanently remove hair.

Hair around nipples? Breast-area skin is sensitive and can't tolerate depilatories, waxing, electrolysis, or shaving. Use sharp clippers to snip away individual hairs.

Leg hair can be removed in several ways: by waxing, depilatories, or shaving. Waxed legs remain relatively hair-free for four to six weeks, but you'll need at least two to three weeks' growth of *new* hair before you can repeat the process. Depilatories leave legs smooth for several days, but may be too irritating for some skins (especially black skin). Shaving is the fastest, easiest, cheapest way to remove leg hair, but most women need to shave every day or so to prevent unsightly stubble.

CLOSE SHAVES

Underarms: Shave when skin and hairs are thoroughly wet. Lather a moisturizing beauty bar and spread foam liberally over underarm area. Using a sharp razor blade, stroke lightly over skin (don't scrape). *Don't* apply deodorant or antiperspirant immediately after shaving—wait at least two hours to prevent irritation. Pat a little cornstarch powder onto underarm area to soothe skin and keep it dry.

Legs: Shave at night, not in the morning. Fluids that accumulate overnight can make your skin "puffy," and you won't get a close shave. A too-long tub soak can puff skin up too, so shave legs after spending just a few minutes in the bath.

Smooth a foaming or gel shave cream over damp legs (gels allow the razor to "glide" over skin more easily than do foams). Easily irritated skin? Opt for a product formulated for sensitive skin (look for ones containing aloe or chamomile).

Shaving *against* hair growth, use long light strokes along calves and thighs, rinsing the razor blade frequently. Shave in a diagonal direction along shinbones to prevent nicks. Use short, feathery strokes around knees and ankles.

Rinse legs well, then pat dry. Soothe just-shaved skin by dusting with baby powder or smoothing on a light moisture lotion.

Avoid swimming in salt water or chlorinated pools for several hours after shaving—salt and chlorine can irritate shaved skin.

> *Prefer the convenience of an* electric razor? *Be sure to use on completely* dry *legs (dust legs with baby powder* before *shaving to reduce friction and discomfort). Shave against the grain of the hair, and avoid "dragging" razor over skin.*
>
> *Electric razors are generally less irritating than safety razors and aren't as likely to cause cuts and nicks. But,* they don't give as close a shave.

PREVENTING INGROWN HAIRS

Women with curly hair (African-American women in particular) are prone to ingrown hairs (the hair curls back into the skin, creating a painful bump). Shaving and waxing can increase the likelihood of ingrown hairs. To help prevent them, use a loofah or polyester facial sponge during your shower or bath to gently abrade dead skin, where hairs tend to get trapped. Shaving legs downward, in the direction of natural hair growth, will also help keep ingrown hairs to a minimum.

SKIN PERFECTERS

Q. What's the best way to camouflage—or get rid

172

of—"spider" veins on the legs?

A. Spider veins are small blood vessels near the skin's surface that have become so enlarged they're visible. They can appear anywhere on the legs and feet, but usually crop up in the knee and upper thigh areas. Some people are genetically predisposed to spider veins—but sun damage is also a common cause. Crossing your legs can aggravate the condition.

You can conceal spider veins with opaque leg makeup (choose a waterproof formula that exactly matches the color of skin on your legs). Because self-tanning lotions darken the skin, they can make spider veins less noticeable.

A dermatologist can inject spider veins with a sclerosing agent (such as hypertonic saline), causing the vessels to collapse. Eventually, the red vein turns a whitish shade.

Q. What are seborrheic keratoses and what's the best way to have them removed?

A. These are raised waxy spots that can appear anywhere on the body, but generally occur on the back, chest, and inner arms. Some are flesh-colored, while others are an unsightly brownish black (they're often mistaken for moles but can grow to an inch or larger in diameter).

Seborrheic keratoses are age-related (you may discover a few during your early forties), and people with oily skin are more apt to develop these usually harmless lesions.

A dermatologist can use liquid nitrogen to freeze, then remove, the bumps. Or they can be scraped off by the doctor, using a straight blade.

Q. Can skin tags be easily removed?

A. These small, flesh-colored or light-brown growths "hang" from the body by a fine stalk (they look like mini-mushrooms). Skin tags can appear anywhere on the body and tend to run in families. Pregnant women are especially prone to developing them.

Many women have skin tags removed for cosmetic reasons, or because they're constantly irritated (by a garment that chafes, for instance), when they appear in the armpit (hampering shaving), or if they in-

Use gentle laundry detergent on clothing—make certain it's completely rinsed away. Harsh detergent residue on clothes (and sheets) can irritate skin, trigger rashes and itching. Some sensitive skins can't tolerate fabric softener sheets (the kind used in dryers). Skip fabric softener if your skin is on the fussy side.

173

terfere with makeup application (tags commonly occur on the eyelids).

A dermatologist can quickly snip off a skin tag, or
remove tags by using electrosurgery (the tag is scraped
off with a special instrument, then an electric needle is
used to "burn" away the base of the area that's been
scraped).

SKIN CHECKUP

According to the Skin Cancer Foundation, skin

BREAST CHECK

Experts estimate that one out of nine women
will develop breast cancer during her lifetime.
Caught early, breast cancer *can* be cured. To
protect yourself, have your gynecologist do a
manual breast exam every year. The American
Cancer Society recommends that asymptomatic
women (and those not in a breast-cancer risk
group*) who are 35 to 39 have *one* baseline
mammogram. Asymptomatic women 40 to 49
should have a mammogram every one or two years.
Asymptomatic women over age 50 should have a
mammogram every year.

Be sure to examine your breasts carefully every
month with these easy self-exam how-to's. (Check
breasts one week after your period, when breasts
usually aren't tender or swollen. If you've had a
hysterectomy, or have gone through menopause,
check breasts the first day of each month.):

· Lie flat on your back, with your left arm
behind your head (place a folded towel under
left shoulder). Using the flat part of fingers on
your right hand, start at the base of your left
breast and work in a series of circular motions (around the breast) in toward the
nipple. Be sure to cover the entire breast.
Press firmly. Feel the area between the breast
and armpit, as well as the armpit itself. Repeat
process on right breast, using left hand. Then,
squeeze the nipple of each breast. If any

Real Beauty . . . Real Women

cancer afflicts more people than any other form of cancer—more than 600,000 new cases are currently diagnosed in the U.S. each year. With early detection and treatment, almost all forms of skin cancer are curable. You, and everyone in your family, can protect yourself by examining your skin from head to toe at least twice a year. (It's a good idea to have a dermatologist check for skin cancers once a year as well.) Examine all parts of your body, including your scalp and the soles of your feet (you may need to use a magnifying mirror for hard-to-see areas. Ask your hairstylist or a friend to check your scalp). Here's what to look for:

liquid appears, report it to your doctor immediately.

· Stand in front of a full-length mirror with your arms at your sides. Look for any irregularities in the shape of breasts as well as for puckering or dimpling of the skin. Clasp hands behind your head and repeat inspection. Press hands on hips, elbows out, checking for irregularities.

· You may find it's easier to examine your breasts while showering. Press fingers against breast and move them over every part as described above.

· Should you find a lump, thickening, dimpling, or discharge from your nipple, report it to your doctor immediately.

*The American Cancer Society suggests you consult your physician regarding frequency of mammograms *if* you fall into one of the following risk categories (your doctor may suggest that you have a baseline mammogram earlier than age 35, or mammograms more frequently during your late thirties and forties):
  You're over the age of 50.
  You have a personal or family history of breast cancer.
  You've never had children, or had your first child after the age of 30.

175

·A skin growth that increases in size and looks pearly, translucent, tan, brown, black, or multi-colored.

·A mole, birthmark, or "beauty mark" that becomes larger or thicker, changes in texture, or has an irregular outline.

·A spot or scab that continues to itch, hurt, crust, scab, erode, or bleed.

·An open sore or wound that doesn't heal or persists for more than four weeks.

If you notice any of the above on *your* skin, schedule a checkup with your doctor or a dermatologist.

BEAUTY WRAP-UP

1. After bathing or showering, mist spray-on bath oil onto damp skin, or smooth on a rich lotion or cream.

2. Opt for bath and shower water that's comfortably warm, not hot. Hot water will leave skin parched.

3. During the winter months, set the thermostat at 68 degrees. Higher temperatures will rob skin of moisture, leave it dry and itchy.

4. To stay dry and fresh, use a *combination* antiperspirant/deodorant and apply on absolutely dry skin for maximum effectiveness.

5. If you have curly hair it's likely you're prone to "ingrowns." Whether you shave or wax your legs, use a loofah or body "scrub" to gently slough away dry skin that can trap curled-back hairs.

6. Twice a year, do a skin-cancer check, looking for any suspicious growths, or changes in moles, birthmarks, or beauty marks.

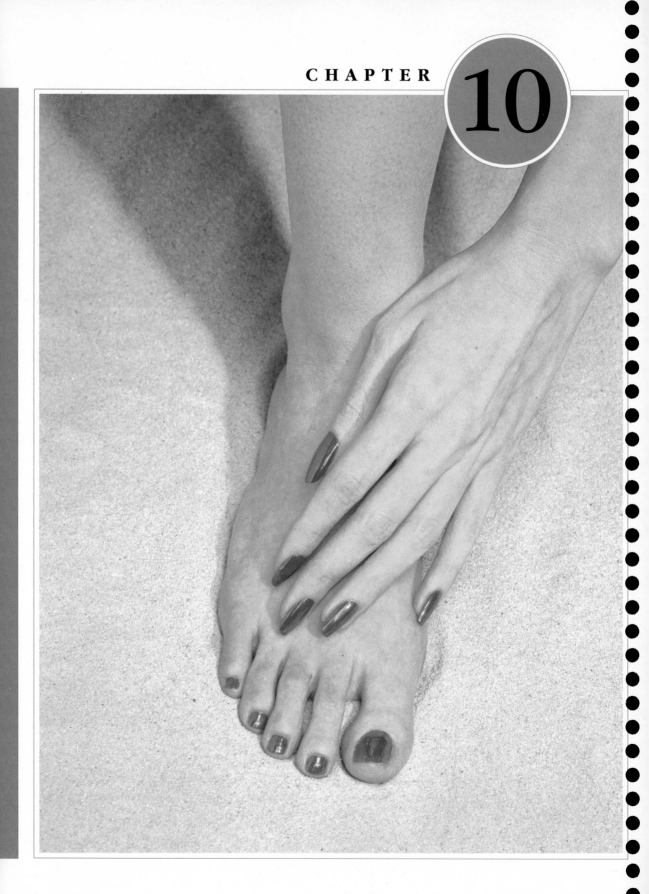

CHAPTER 10

Once a week, treat yourself to a manicure. Below, step-by-step how-to's for "professional" results:

TIP-TOP TIPS

1. Wash your hands with a moisturizing soap, then massage a rich cream over hands, paying special attention to cuticles.

2. Remove old polish, using cotton balls soaked in non-acetone polish remover (to guard against the drying effects of remover, mix a mini-drop of olive or baby oil into 1 teaspoon of remover). Avoid *rubbing* nails—you can actually strip away the top layer, leaving nails dry, prone to splitting. Instead, gently press cotton against nail for several seconds, then sweep from base to tip.

3. Using an emery board, gently file nails in one direction only, on underside of nail (filing tops can cause splitting). The center of the nail should be square or oval, the corners gently rounded (see "Short or Long?" below).

4. Soften cuticles by soaking in warm water for 5 minutes (add several drops of baby or bath oil to water).

T.L.C. for Hands and Feet

5. Pat hands and nails dry and apply a gentle cuticle softener around entire cuticle; leave on for 2 to 3 minutes. Wrap tip of an orange stick in cotton; dip tip in olive oil. Use to gently push back cuticles (don't push back too far—you'll risk infection or injury to the nail). Rinse off oil and cuticle cream.

6. Use cuticle scissors to *carefully* snip hangnails (avoid cutting actual cuticles).

7. If cuticles are very rough, gently file with the smooth side of a "buffing" emery board. Massage a rich cream over hands and into cuticles.

8. Use a damp cloth to wipe hand cream off nails and pat dry.

9. Stroke on one layer of base coat (choose an antistain product if your nails are prone to yellowing, an antipeeling base coat if nails are weak, a ridge-filling formula if nails are ridged or "pitted"). Allow to dry for at least 2 minutes.

10. Apply first coat of nail enamel in three neat strokes. Begin with your little finger. Brush up center of nail from cuticle to tip. Then, once up each side. Allow to dry for 2 minutes. Repeat application. Let dry 2 minutes. (Note: Don't pick up too much polish with brush—you'll end up with uneven ridges of color.)

11. Stroke on top coat in same way you applied enamel. Let nails dry for 30 minutes to prevent smudging. To quick-dry, dip fingertips in ice water for 10 seconds, or set your hair dryer on "cool" and, holding nozzle 8 inches from fingers, aim air at tips for 60 seconds for each hand.

SHORT OR LONG?

Short nails are best for "active fingers," professional-looking, and a good bet for less-than-perfect nails. The nail tip and fingertip should meet (or have nail length no more than 1/8 inch beyond fingertip).

Average-length nails are a smart choice for career women and are best for nails that are healthy and smooth. The nail tip should extend 1/4 inch beyond the tip of your finger.

Long nails are more eye-catching than fashionable these days and are best suited for special occasions. The nail tip should extend no more than 1/3 inch beyond the fingertip.

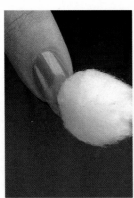
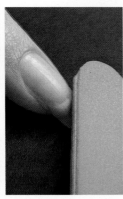
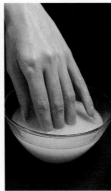
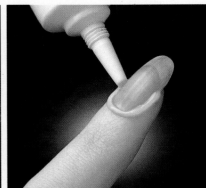

Real Beauty . . . Real Women

NAIL MENDERS

Chipped polish? Don't remove enamel. Instead, stroke enamel over chipped area only and allow to dry. Then, smooth enamel over *entire* nail, from base to tip. Let dry. Stroke on top coat.

Split or torn nail? Keep nail-mending tape on hand (paper, linen, and silk are best). Tear off tape to the length of split, plus 1/8 inch beyond nail's tip. Press self-sticking tape onto clean nail and tuck excess under tip (or apply nail glue to tear and place nail tape on top). Gently file to smooth. Brush on base coat, enamel, and top coat to finish. Mended nails need a layer of top coat added each day for extra protection—and a smooth, glossy look.

No mending tape? In a pinch, repair your nail with instant-bonding glue and a piece of tea-bag or coffee-filter paper. Remove old polish and gently file nail top to create a slightly rough surface. Smooth on a dab of glue. Using just enough tea-bag or coffee-filter material to cover the tear, place on nail. Dot on a little more glue; let dry, then file to smooth. Apply base coat, enamel, and top coat.

Finished your manicure only to smudge one nail? To avoid getting polish remover on other nails, use the knuckles of your index and middle fingers to grip a cotton ball and moisten it with remover. Wipe over smudged nail and re-do enamel. Just a tiny smudge on one nail? Use the pad of your index finger to dab a hint of remover over smudged area (use a super-light touch). Let dry, then apply a coat of enamel.

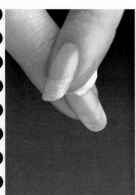
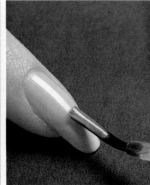
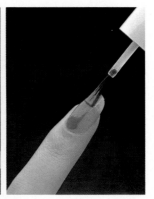

No time for an entire manicure? Try doing a few steps at a time. At night, follow "Tip-Top Tips" steps through application of first coat of enamel. The next morning, apply a second coat of enamel. Later that day, stroke on top coat. (This will allow plenty of drying time between coats.)

RX FOR PROBLEM NAILS

Horizontal ridges can result from "rough manicures" (using an orange stick or cuticle pusher to force cuticles back), as well as certain illnesses and improper nutrition. *Cure:* Be sure your diet is well-balanced (your doctor may suggest you take an all-purpose daily multivitamin). Use a ridge-filling base coat and buff nails weekly to smooth.

Soft, weak nails are often inherited (Asian women sometimes have soft, "bendable" nails), but crash diets can also trigger peeling and weakening. *Cure:* Patch damaged areas and use a nail hardener for extra protection. Leave old polish on while filing to prevent splits and tears. Avoid extreme low-calorie diets.

Dry, brittle nails are frequently caused by exposure to household cleansers and harsh soaps, dipping hands in and out of water, plus too-frequent use of nail-polish remover. As you age, your nails tend to become drier, but dry nails can also signal vitamin A or calcium deficiency or thyroid disease. *Cure:* Wear rubber gloves for all household chores. Apply hand cream several times daily and opt for nail-strengthening creams and base coats. Use an oily polish remover—and change polish once a week maximum. (To avoid remover altogether, try the new "peel-off" nail enamels.)

Yellow nails and yellow tips are often caused by the pigments in darker-toned nail enamels. Yellow nails can also be a warning sign of circulatory problems (poor circulation slows nail growth, producing thicker, rougher, yellow-tinted nails). Beta-carotene supplements and the antibiotic tetracycline can also cause yellowing. *Cure:* If your hands frequently feel cold, be sure to have your doctor check for a circulatory disor-

182

der. Using a buffing file, gently smooth over nails to slightly remove stain. Or, rub fresh lemon over nails to bleach. Always use base coat under polish to *prevent* staining, or use two layers of base coat, or a ridge-filler topped with base coat. Very yellow nails? Take a break from polish for two to three weeks, buffing nails daily to keep them glossy.

To lighten *tips*, wrap cotton around the end of an orange stick and moisten with hydrogen peroxide. Run along underside of nail.

Vertical ridges can indicate circulatory diseases such as rheumatoid arthritis, but are often caused by too-vigorous manicures. *Cure:* Once a physical problem has been ruled out, gently "file" tops of nails with a "buffing board" to smooth, then use ridge-filler base coat.

Orange-brown or brownish-black nails often result from exposure to hydroquinone (in skin-bleaching creams) and paraphenylenediamine (a chemical in hair dyes). *Cure:* Buff nails nightly to gradually remove the stain. Wear latex (rubber) gloves when applying skin bleaches and hair dyes.

White spots on nails usually result from trauma (over-zealous manicures). Totally opaque, white, or half-white nails may be hereditary or caused by vitamin deficiency or certain illnesses. *Cure:* Let your doctor examine your nails to rule out illness. Use white-toned ridge-filler base coat to help even out color, then apply a medium-dark enamel.

Separation of nail from nail bed is your cue to see a dermatologist. Fungal infections, diabetes, psoriasis, and many other disorders can trigger separation. *Cure:* Keep your hands out of water as much as possible; fungal infections thrive in a moist environment.

Note: Because your nails can say a lot about your health—signaling certain illnesses or nutritional deficiencies—let your doctor take a look at your *bare* nails during your yearly physical exam.

DID YOU KNOW . . .

·that it takes three to six months for an entirely

183

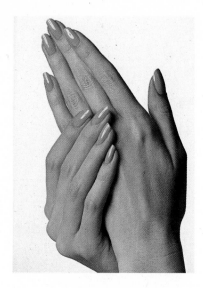

new nail to form?

· that the average growth of a nail is 1/8 inch per month?

· that the middle fingernail grows the fastest and the thumbnail is the "snail of nails"?

· that if you're right-handed, nails will grow faster on your right hand (and the reverse if you're a lefty)?

· that "active" fingers—ones that are frequently stimulated by piano-playing, typing—experience the most rapid nail growth?

· that nails grow faster during warm weather?

· that the most rapid nail growth occurs during pregnancy?

FASHIONABLE FINGERTIPS

Your nail enamel should complement your makeup (blush, lipstick) and clothing; all should be in the same color family. If your skin tone is pinky-blue, or if you're wearing "cool" shades of clothing, opt for cool or blue-based nail colors in pinks, mauves, wines, plums. If your skin is yellow- or golden-based or when you wear "warm" shades of clothing, choose warm colors for your fingertips, like peaches, corals, and browns.

Change of Season, Change of Climate

Spring, summer, and warmer climates call for lighter, brighter nails. Opt for warm corals, peaches, and oranges, or cool pinks, mauves, and opalescents. Semi-frosted shades give nails an "airy" look during the summer.

In the *fall, winter, and colder areas*, choose rich creamy nail colors in burnished coppers and berries,

184

mauves, wines, and deep garnet reds. Stroke frosts and opalescent shades over a cream color to add sparkle for holiday and evening looks.

Professional Tips

Your nail length and color should complement your career.

Field	Nail Fashion
Medical, diet/health care, day-care center, restaurant	Shorter or average-length nails. French manicure, clear or nude enamel, for a clean, healthy look.
Financial or legal environment, executive office, politics, school	Shorter or average-length nails. For a professional touch, neutral shades like soft mauves, pink, warm peaches, honey.
Office, retail, fashion, factory, or creative environment	Choose a length most comfortable for you. Opt for classic red or fashion shades to match your outfit.
Hands-on careers: repair, installation, arts, crafts, musician	Short, clean nails are a must. If you opt for color, polish nails with clear enamel or nude polish—they're easiest to keep neat, fix quickly if they chip.

Fast French Manicure

1. Do your basic manicure and apply clear base coat. Let dry 2 minutes.

2. Brush creamy white or neutral beige enamel onto nail tip only. (Stroke brush across tip, following natural line of nail, in one smooth sweep.) Let dry 2 minutes.

3. Apply sheer pink or clear enamel over entire nail—two coats for a more protective, glossier finish. Let each coat dry 2 minutes. Apply top coat.

HANDS-ON BEAUTY

Wear gloves or mittens in cold weather to keep hands from drying out. Smooth a rich cream onto hands before donning gloves. The warmth from the gloves will "seal" cream into skin.

If you must wash your hands frequently, use soap on the palms of hands and bottoms of fingers only. Soap and water (especially the harsh kind in public restrooms) strip moisture from the thin skin on top of hands, soak right through nail polish to dry out nails.

If you wash your hair in the kitchen sink (instead of the shower), wear rubber gloves to protect hands, nails, from water, shampoo.

Save your nails by using a pencil to dial rotary telephones. Use pads of fingers to pick up small objects. Rely on a metal nail file to pry open jewelry clasps. Use the eraser end of a pencil to poke around in your handbag. Use your knuckles to ring doorbells, push buttons.

Keep hand cream "handy"—with dispensers in the bathroom, kitchen, bedroom, at work.

PERFECT PEDICURE

1. Use polish remover to whisk away old polish from toenails.

2. Soak feet for 10 to 15 minutes in warm water (add 3 teaspoons bath oil to water to help soften cuticles and rough heels). Dab a rich, thick cream onto a clean pumice stone, then gently rub over rough areas—heels, undersides of toes, sides, and balls of feet.

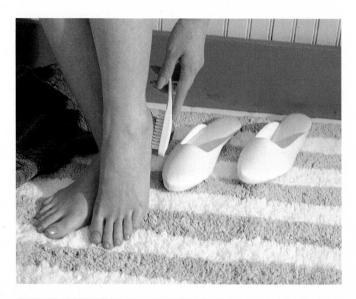

186

3. Use a toenail clipper to trim nails straight across (nails should extend no more than 1/8 inch beyond ends of toes). Using a coarse-textured emery board, file away rough edges and slightly taper corners (don't file or cut nails sharply into corners of toes—you can end up with painful, ingrown toenails).

4. Apply cuticle softener and allow it to soak in for several minutes. Rinse toes, then use a clean orange stick to gently push back cuticles. With cuticle scissors, trim hangnails. Reapply softener and smooth cuticles with a buffer. Rinse feet well.

5. Moisturize and massage feet, using a rich foot or hand cream. Place thumbs on top of your foot near ankle, fingers near heel. Move in circles toward toes. Use thumb and first finger to massage each toe. Clean toenails with cotton or a damp cloth to remove cream.

6. Smooth toenail ridges by buffing gently. Thread a rolled tissue (or foam "toe-spreader") between toes to separate, then stroke on base coat. Allow to dry for 2 minutes.

7. Using nail enamel in a color that matches your fingertips, stroke onto little toe first, brushing up the center from cuticle to tip. Then, quickly stroke color up each side of nail. Allow to dry for 2 minutes, then repeat application.

8. Apply one layer of top coat. Let dry for 30 minutes.

FOOT FIXERS

Treat tired, achy feet to a soothing soak. Use a commercial "foot bath," or pour 2 tablespoons Epsom salts into a large container and soak feet for 10 minutes.

Prevent athlete's foot by thoroughly drying feet (especially between toes) after bathing and swimming. Dust feet liberally with foot or baby powder and opt for cotton or wool socks (synthetic ones trap moisture that allows the fungus that causes athlete's foot to grow). Sandals or shoes made of all-natural materials like leather help feet stay cool, dry, preventing perspiration.

Wear "swimmer's shoes" at pools to avoid the trail

For Long-lasting Manicures and Pedicures

·*After applying top coat, hold brush parallel to tip of nail and sweep top coat slightly under nail to prevent chipping.*

·*Use top coat every other day to keep finger and toe nails looking glossy, help prevent chips.*

T.L.C. for Hands and Feet

of athlete's foot fungi other swimmers leave near the pool and in the locker room. Avoid sharing towels.

If you *do* get athlete's foot, wash and dry your feet thoroughly every day, and apply an antifungal ointment or spray twice daily.

HEEL SUPER-SMOOTHER

Before bedtime, soak feet in warm water for 5 minutes. Pat dry. Mix 1 tablespoon sugar with 1 tablespoon sunflower or grapeseed oil (both are available at grocery and health-food stores). Massage into heel area for 2 minutes, then rinse off. Rub a little more oil onto heels; use tissue to blot up excess. Then don clean thick cotton socks. Sunflower and grapeseed oils are rich sources of essential fatty acids, which provide a superb "moisture barrier" on the skin, softening even the roughest, driest heels.

COSMETIC COST-SAVERS

·If nail enamel thickens, place bottle (screw cap on tightly!) in a cup of very warm water for several minutes.

·Keep polish from getting gooey by storing it in the refrigerator.

·Keep nail polish caps from sticking by smoothing a little petroleum jelly around neck of new bottles. If the bottle is old, wipe the inside of the cap with a cotton swab dampened with nail polish remover.

CROSS-COUNTRY BEAUTY

Do you live in the *Midwest* or extreme *Northeast*? Keep nails and hands from drying out by wearing *thermal-lined* gloves or mittens during the winter. Opt for mittens—in lieu of gloves—whenever possible.

Your fingers "snuggle" together, generating more heat in mittens.

If you live in the *Southwest* or *Southern California*, get in the habit of smoothing sunscreen onto the backs of hands and fingers to prevent sun-related wrinkling, "age" spots, and skin cancer.

Live in a state like *Florida* that allows you to swim almost all year 'round? Smooth a protective top coat onto nails daily to help guard against the drying effects of water and chlorine in pools.

BEAUTY WRAP-UP

1. Avoid using nail-polish remover more than once a week. Used too often, it can leave nails dry and brittle.

2. Opt for shorter rather than longer nails. They'll look sophisticated, professional, and healthy.

3. Keep cuticles neat-looking by using a clean, damp cloth to gently push them back after every shower or bath.

4. Choose nail colors that coordinate with blush and lip shades, complement your wardrobe.

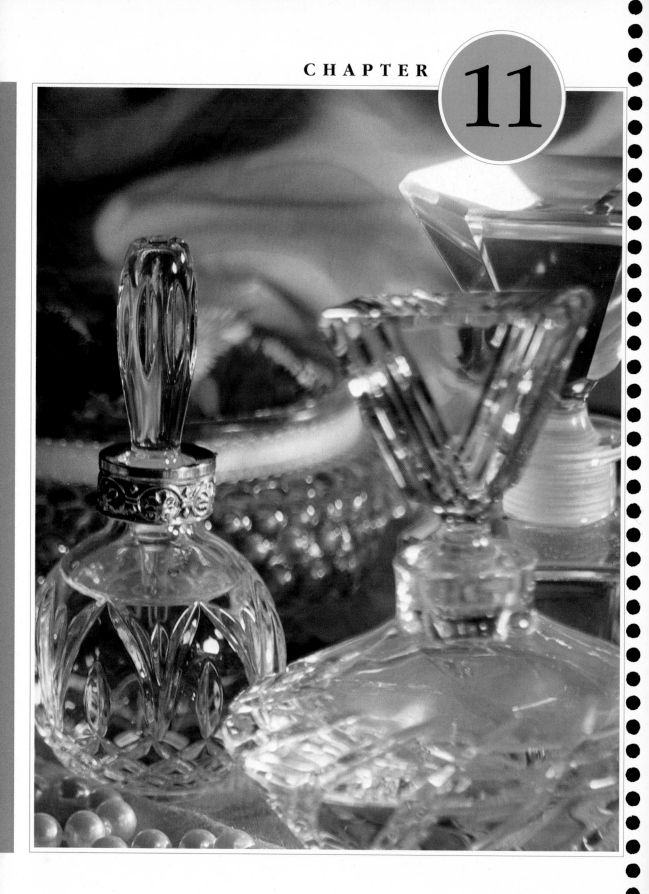

CHAPTER 11

Fragrance, in its many delightful varieties, has always been an important aspect of femininity, sensuality—but today, fragrance has become an absolutely essential part of the modern woman's personality, her special aura of beauty. While perfume was once reserved for "special occasions," and a woman wore one "signature scent," the nineties woman sees her life as a *series* of important moments. She may wear fragrance every day and at night, creating a "wardrobe" of scents that suit her every mood, celebrate her individuality.

FLORAL OR FRUITY? CITRUSY OR SPICY?

Selecting fragrance is a highly personal experience. No fragrance smells exactly the same on everyone—your skin interacts with fragrance to create a unique scent. That's why you can't accurately judge a fragrance when your best friend is wearing it. Sniffing a fragrance from the bottle won't give you a good idea of how it will smell on you either.

To accurately test a fragrance, dab or mist it onto your inner or outer wrist and experience the way it changes during the next 10 to 15 minutes. Your first impression is the "top note." Soon, the full impression of the fragrance will begin to unfold. This stage is referred to as the "middle note" or heart. The full character or long-term impression of a scent isn't discernible until a few minutes after application, when it's had time to blend with the natural oils on your skin. The fragrance is altered by your individual chemistry, providing the missing note—and making the scent distinctly yours alone.

Botanical Beauty

There are six great "families" of fragrance:

· Single Florals
· Floral Bouquets
· Leafy, Woodsy, Mossy Blends
· Spicy, Fruity Blends

191

·Oriental Blends
·Modern Blends

(For a description of each, see "Test Your Fragrance 'Personality'," pages 193-94.)

To discover the family—or families—that are right for you, follow these fragrance-testing tips:

1. Experiment with *many* fragrances to make the best choice.

2. Never try more than three scents at a time (your "nose" will become confused). Try a fragrance on each wrist, another on your forearm.

3. Allow 5 to 10 minutes before smelling to allow the heart of the fragrance to develop.

4. It's best to test fragrance in the afternoon, when your sense of smell is keener, your sinuses are clearer.

5. Don't test fragrance after eating spicy, garlicky, or curried foods—*their* essence can seep through your skin, altering the scent.

6. Once you decide on a particular fragrance, test other scents in the same family group. If you love rose, you may be drawn to other floral aromas, such as gardenia, lily-of-the-valley, honeysuckle, jasmine, lilac.

FRAGRANCE DICTIONARY

Fragrance comes in many forms. Here are the most common:

Liquids. The most traditional form of fragrance is liquid.

Cologne is perfume oil in an alcohol base and is available in varying strengths (some colognes are quite subtle, while the "ultra-colognes" have the greatest impact and are longest-lasting).

Perfume is composed of the highest concentration of perfume oils (often containing hundreds of ingredients). The most expensive of fragrances, perfume is also the longest-lasting.

Toilet water (eau de toilette) is more intense and longer-lasting than cologne, more subtle than per-

192

fume.

Pump Sprays. These are liquid fragrances *(cologne, perfume,* and *toilet water)* that are drawn up through a slender tube and forced out through a small opening at the top. The mist created by a spray covers a wider area of the skin than ordinary liquid fragrances and results in greater diffusion.

Creams. *Creams, lotions,* and *glacé* fragrances take longer to diffuse than liquid forms because the warmth of the skin is needed to "release" the fragrance. Creams are especially convenient for travel (since there's little chance of spillage). They also provide a mild, subtle scent.

Oils. *Perfume oils* are highly concentrated fragrance in an oil base. Extremely long-lasting, they're very intense in aroma.

TEST YOUR FRAGRANCE "PERSONALITY"

Find the description that best fits you, then choose the fragrances that are a perfect match. (You *may* see aspects of your personality in more than one "profile." Lucky you! Enjoy sampling a multitude of fragrances.)

Personality Profile

1. You're upbeat, energetic. When you wake up in the morning, you know there's *nothing* you can't do if you set your mind to it. Life is truly a banquet, and you eagerly look forward to new opportunities. Whether you're twenty or sixty, people see you as "youthful."

2. You are blessed with a lyrical, poetic bent—often slipping into a fantasy world of daydreams. People describe you as "creative." You think of yourself as romantic and your wardrobe reflects your personality, with fluid, draped dresses in Monet pastels.

3. You love all things beautiful and crave sensual pleasures—the feel of silk and cashmere against your skin, the heady scent of fresh-cut flowers in your home. A walk through the garden restores you in body and mind.

4. You're inventive, enterprising, bold. You prefer clothes that are classic—tailored, but softly feminine, blouses and suits, and, for evening, a simple black dress and a string of pearls.

5. Happy-go-lucky and social by nature, you adore parties—in fact, being with people is your favorite pastime. Your clothes are just a bit on the trendy side, and your friends follow your lead when it comes to fashion.

6. You're sophisticated and sexy (or, so says your partner!). *You* know that you prefer mystery and drama (you love the opera), and you choose clothes and makeup in deep, sumptuous jewel tones, like garnet, jade, and sapphire.

7. You're active and love the outdoors, into health foods and fitness. Independent, visionary, you'd like to save the world (or, at the very least, clean up the environment). "Natural" cosmetics appeal to you, and you opt for makeup in subtle, but rich, earth tones.

8. You love to travel (if only in your dreams) and long to visit exotic places like Africa, Japan, and India. You've seen *Murder on the Orient Express* at least four times, and your idea of the perfect mini-vacation is a "mystery weekend" at an old Victorian inn.

Fragrance Families

Each personality type has two ideal fragrances.

A. *Single florals* capture the essence of a single blossom like rose, jasmine, carnation, gardenia.

B. *Floral bouquets* blend a bouquet of different flower notes into an intricate and subtle harmony. You may not be able to identify the specific flowers, but the fragrance is definitely "flowery" in character.

C. *Leafy, woodsy, mossy blends* combine aromatic woods, like cedar, with the aromas of flower stems, leaves, ferns, oakmoss, and other herbal scents for a clean, refreshing fragrance.

D. *Spicy, fruity blends* meld the clean, fresh quality of citrus fruits and pungent spices, such as clove, cinnamon, or ginger, with spicy flower aromas, such as carnation, and hints of mellow peach-like warmth. These are apt to be sparkling, outdoorsy fragrances—

light and fresh—but they may evolve into rich, full-bodied scents.

E. *Oriental blends* evoke the mystery and richness of the Orient through sophisticated combinations of musk and amber, along with many exotic blossoms. These blends are apt to be haunting, intense, and sweet or smoky.

F. *Modern blends* may contain notes from any or all other fragrance categories, yet they do not duplicate anything in nature. Rather, they're dazzling new creations of the perfumer. They have a full-bodied total impact that is characterized by a brilliant sparkle.

Which do you think go together? Guess.

Answers:

(1) D, F; (2) A, B; (3) B, E; (4) A, F; (5) D, F; (6) B, E; (7) D, C; (8) C, E.

"LAYERING" SCENTS MAKES SENSE

Once you've chosen a scent, use that fragrance in its many forms to "surround yourself" with a subtle veil of scent. By "layering" a fragrance you intensify its impact, extend its staying power for hours.

Using products in the same fragrance family, begin with a perfumed soap and matching bath oil. Follow with body lotion and talc in the same scent. Then, lightly mist or dab on cologne and perfume. Freshen fragrance a few times throughout the day (carry a purse-size spray in your handbag).

How to apply cologne and perfume?

·Splash or spray *cologne* onto body, neck, arms, and legs after bathing to create a "base" for perfume.
·Stroke *perfume* onto any of the "pulse points": temples, behind ears, base of throat, nape of neck, over collarbone, inside elbows, onto backs of wrists, inside of wrists, backs of knees, backs of ankles. The heat from these pulse points intensifies a fragrance's impact.

195

SCENTS FOR SUMMER

Warm temperatures turn up a fragrance's intensity. Opt for a lighter scent in a subtle form, like cologne, for day wear. Save perfume for evening.

If you prefer a *very* delicate aura of scent, use fragranced body lotion in lieu of cologne during the day. Or, let scented soap and bath oil enfold you in a fragrant veil.

Planning to spend time in the sun? Fragrance can interact with the sun's rays, triggering a photosensitivity reaction (rash, redness). Rather than applying fragrance directly onto skin, lightly mist your beach cover-up with cologne, or tuck a handkerchief scented with your favorite fragrance into a pocket.

MORE "SCENTSATIONAL" TIPS

Create a "fragrance wardrobe" to express your various moods, complement your many fashion looks. Choose three or four fragrances from different families, such as floral bouquet, Oriental, or spicy-fruity blends.

Remember that fragrance rises. If you apply scent behind your ears only, *you* won't enjoy the full impact. Be sure to mist or dab onto wrists, insides of elbows, behind knees.

Don't try to achieve an entire day's worth of fragrance power by "mega-dosing" in the morning. The result can be stifling (and offensive to others!). Instead, carry perfume or cologne in your purse and reapply fragrance during the day.

Switch fragrances periodically. If you wear one scent for too long, your "nose" will tire of it.

If you love a particular fragrance but find that it doesn't work well with your body chemistry, lightly mist the scent onto a cotton pad or handkerchief and conceal it in a jacket or skirt pocket.

Avoid letting cologne or perfume spray "mist down" onto clothing (particularly silk). The alcohol content can damage fine fabrics. Apply fragrance *before* dressing—or cover your clothing with an old shirt before spritzing on scent.

196

Avoid exposing fragrances to extreme cold or heat or light. All can spoil the scent's delicate balance.

Opt for fragrance-free or "natural"-smelling hairsprays. Heavily fragranced sprays can interfere with your cologne or perfume.

SURROUND YOURSELF WITH BOTANICAL DELIGHTS

Extend the pleasures of fragrance to every facet of your life with these sweet suggestions:

Place vases of fresh-cut flowers or pots of flowering plants throughout the house during the spring and early summer. Choose flowers or plants with vivid, long-lasting perfumes for hallways and entryways. A potted hyacinth or small bouquet of freesia will perfume a large area—let its scent waft from the entryway throughout your home (these intensely aromatic flowers may be overpowering in a dining room or living room).

During the fall and winter, when fresh flowers aren't readily available, opt for bowls of fragrant fruits, like ripe apples and pears. Or, lightly mist a floral or woodsy scent over bunches of dried flowers, herbs, silk flower arrangements.

Place bowls of potpourri throughout the house. (If you have small children or curious pets, make sure potpourri is well out of their reach!) Buy potpourri—or make your own from dried rose petals.

On holidays, keep a pot of "simmering spices" on the stove. Stud a small orange with 12 to 20 cloves. Heat 3 cups water to boiling, then reduce to a slow simmer. Add the orange pomander to water, along with 2 cinnamon sticks and a dash of nutmeg. The spicy fragrance will serve as a delicious welcome to guests.

Use "home fragrance sprays" (more subtle and elegant than room fresheners) for ambience. Dust scented "carpet powder" onto rugs, then vacuum up.

For special occasions, light scented candles in the bathroom, bedroom, guest powder room.

Saturate a cotton ball with scented bath oil and

hide it in a decorative vase or bowl to secretly scent the bathroom, living room, bedroom.

Tuck sachets in among sheets and towels in a linen closet, as well as into lingerie drawers.

Perfume or cologne losing its "punch"? Use the last few sprays in lieu of room freshener.

Tuck unwrapped perfumed guest soaps into your luggage before storing. The bags will smell delicious, not musty, the next time you pack for a trip.

Attach sachets to coat hangers in your closet, or opt for covered scented hangers.

Use scented paper to line clothing drawers. Or use scented paper fragrance samples. (You can make your own by misting your favorite fragrance onto white blotter paper.)

Mist stationery, cards, with your favorite scent before sending to a special friend (or sweetheart!).

One large Japanese corporation is currently putting aromachology findings to the test—pumping certain fragrances into the workplace to reduce stress and promote worker performance. Researchers at the renowned Memorial-Sloan Kettering Cancer Center, in New York City, have used heliotropin to significantly reduce anxiety in patients undergoing stressful medical procedures such as MRI (magnetic resonance imaging) scans.

CROSS-COUNTRY BEAUTY

For fun, match your fragrance to your area of the U.S.

Pacific Northwest cities like *Seattle* and *Portland* stay lush and green all year 'round, and it's likely you take advantage of this natural paradise, hiking, mountain-climbing, camping. Choose a woodsy-mossy scent, with hints of sandalwood, rosewood, cedar, and earthy oakmoss and fern notes, creating a clean, crisp, "foresty" fragrance.

Live in an exotic city like *New Orleans*? Look for a sultry, mysterious Oriental fragrance that combines brilliant exotic flowers and herbs.

If you're from a strong, powerful city like *Chicago*

THE SCIENCE OF SCENT

The ancients practiced "aromatherapy," using fragrant oils and herbs in body massage and therapeutic baths. Today, moderns at exclusive spas, skin-care salons, and "scent boutiques" use aromatherapy techniques to heal, beautify, and soothe the body and mind.

Not so long ago, scientists were apt to turn up their noses at aromatherapy, viewing it as "just another New Age trend." But in recent years, independent research and university studies have been proving the amazing "power of scent." There's even a new "science of scent," *aromachology*, developed by the Fragrance Research Fund, and researchers worldwide are studying how scent affects the psyche. Here's what they've found:

· Certain substances in nutmeg and valerian oils seem to reduce stress in humans.

· Lavender oil has a mild sedative effect.

· Odors appear to alter mood or even reduce depression. (In clinical studies, depressed patients were given "odor therapy" by two different methods. In one method, scents— floral, fruity, and food odors—were piped into each patient's room. In a second trial, patients sniffed the scents from open bottles. Mood improvement was seen clinically—and in depression-scale tests—after patients were exposed to the odors.)

· Jasmine seems to have a stimulating effect.

· A combination of peppermint and muguet (lily-of-the-valley) help improve task performance and may be valuable in job-related settings.

· Use of fragrance may heighten a sense of self-esteem and confidence.

· The sense of smell functions even during sleep, and jasmine and peppermint tend to waken people and may have potential as "odorant alarm clocks," while heliotropin (a sweet vanilla-like odor) slightly enhances sleep.

199

or *New York*, try a vibrant, sparkling modern blend with a rich top note.

If you hail from the South, where every porch has half a dozen hanging baskets overflowing with flowers and bouquets fill every room of the house with fragrance, choose a floral scent with a flamboyant touch of magnolia (which is actually a blend of jasmine, neroli, rose, and ylang-ylang).

BEAUTY WRAP-UP

1. Don't limit yourself to one scent. Instead, create a "wardrobe" of three or four fragrances to suit your every mood, to complement your various fashion looks.

2. Don't judge a fragrance by the way it smells on someone else. Perfumes and colognes interact with *your* body chemistry to create a highly unique and individual scent.

3. After dabbing scent onto your wrist, wait 5 to 10 minutes before smelling to allow the heart of the fragrance to evolve.

4. "Layer" fragrance—from scented soaps and bath oils to colognes and perfumes—to give scent staying power.

5. Apply scent to pulse points, like the insides of elbows, backs and insides of wrists, backs of knees. The warmth generated in these areas will intensify a fragrance's impact.

6. Surround yourself with botanical delights by filling your home with bouquets of fresh-cut flowers or bowls of potpourri. Tuck sachets into lingerie drawers and linen cupboards. Light scented candles in the living room, bedroom, guest bath to create ambience on special occasions.

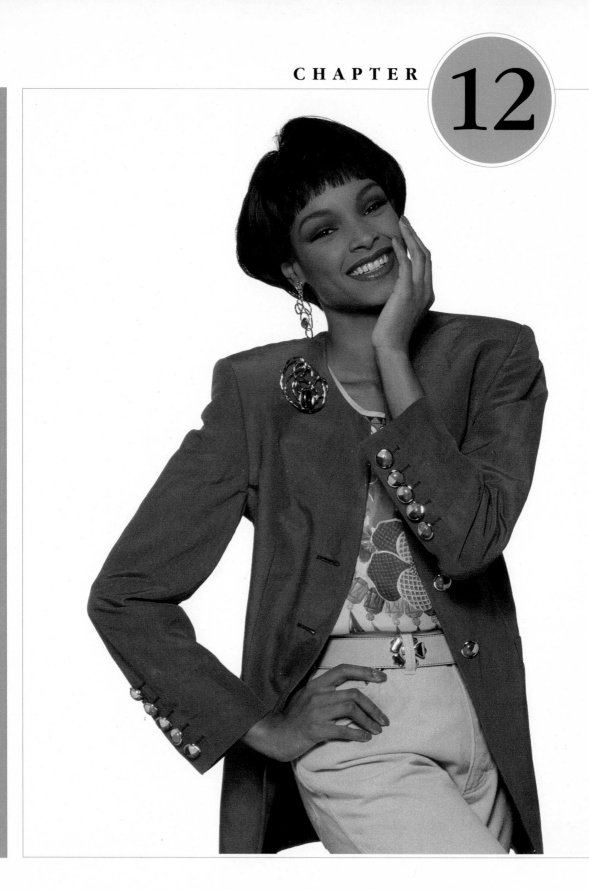

CHAPTER 12

Accessories are, perhaps, the most important part of your total fashion look (and, because they can be used like cosmetics to give warmth and glow to your complexion, a "beauty must" as well). The right accessories are smart money-savers too; they'll outlast your clothes by years, and well-chosen earrings, necklaces, pins, belts, and scarves allow you to transform a wardrobe of just a few basics into dozens of different and exciting looks that are uniquely *you*.

ACCESSORY KNOW-HOW

Choose jewelry, scarves, belts that are well-made. Look for quality pieces. (You *don't* have to buy *real* gold or silver, or authentic pearls, emeralds, sapphires, or diamonds—but *do* make certain costume jewelry *looks* expensive, even if you paid bargain prices!)

Accessories should complement your body size. If you're petite and small-boned, beware of too-big or too-bold necklaces, earrings, and scarves that may overwhelm you. Stick with smaller, more discreet pieces.

Big-boned? You can carry off bolder accessories, big square-cut scarves, larger pins, dramatic necklaces and earrings. Tiny pieces of jewelry will get "lost" on you.

Add-Ons That Add Up to a Great Look

·Tailor your accessories to fit the season. Heavier gold and silver items, like "cuff" bracelets and thick chain-link necklaces, add richness to fall and winter fashions. In the summer, switch to lighter, airier pieces, like a wristful of super-skinny bangles, or natural wooden or faux ivory beads, or earrings and necklaces in a delicate mix of silver and turquoise, gold and coral.

·Invest in one or two "trendy" items. An unusual pin or art deco or sixties print scarf can update more conservative blazers, dresses, sweaters.

CLEVER PROBLEM-SOLVERS
Body Shapers

If you're petite, or your figure's on the round side, you can look taller and slimmer by wearing a long necklace (look for "opera length" pearls, 28 to 30 inches, or a lengthy chain studded with rhinestones or multicolored stones, or a super-long silver or gold chain with a decorative pendant). Another slenderizer: an oblong scarf.

Heavy hips? Opt for small, thin bracelets—or none at all. A bracelet can call attention to the hip area. Instead, choose big lapel pins, a short, striking necklace or choker, bold earrings, or a colorful scarf, knotted at the throat—anything to direct attention *upward*.

Thick waist? If you *do* wear belts, choose ones that are 3/4 inch or less, and avoid eye-catching buckles. Belt color should blend with the color of your skirt, slacks, or dress to avoid "cutting you in half."

Short-waisted? Choose a skinny belt that buckles loosely, forming a slight "V" shape to give the illusion of a longer-waisted look. Belt color should match the color of your blouse or sweater to create an impression of length.

Face Shapers

To slim a round face, select jewelry shapes that cause the eye to move vertically. Rectangular, square, diamond-shaped, or drop earrings and pins are a smart choice. Earrings with vertical lines or stripes are good face-slimmers too. V-shaped jewelry will slim a moon face; if you wear a choker, it should form a V or include a square, diamond, or rectangular pendant.

To add width to a long, thin face, opt for rounder jewelry shapes or those that cause the eye to move horizontally. Round, crescent, domed, or swirled earrings are most flattering, and short necklaces or chokers will help shorten your face.

Soften a square face with jewelry pieces that are gently rounded at the edges (avoid square or horizontal shapes). Choose round or oval earrings and pins. Circular chokers and round shapes at the throat soften the jawline. V-shaped necklaces are a flattering option.

Droopy jowls? Avoid dangling earrings—they'll "pull" your face down even more. Instead, choose earrings that sit high on the lobe. Shapes with a point or detailing at the top (inverted "V's", or "king's crowns") will direct attention upward.

BALANCING ACT

Jewelry placement involves four primary focal points: ears, neck, shoulders, and wrist. Too much or too little in any of these areas looks awkward or "unfinished."

· If you wear a pin on the left shoulder, try a bracelet on the right wrist, or vice versa.

· When you wear a necklace *and* pin, each should be simple. The necklace should be longer rather than short to avoid clutter at the throat area.

· Earrings should provide a balanced, finished look, even with the most casual clothes. Unless you're very big-boned, stick with this rule of thumb: If you wear large, bold earrings, keep other accessories—pins, necklaces—small. If you go with smaller earrings, opt for a bigger, more dramatic necklace or pin. (Large, big-boned, or tall women can carry off multiples of dramatic pieces.)

DETAILS MAKE THE DIFFERENCE

Beautiful jewelry and richly textured and patterned scarves can warm, brighten your complexion.

When "Less" Isn't Enough

Create impact with multiples. A tiny lapel pin or a single gold bangle at the wrist can get lost. Try randomly placing four to six little lapel pins on your blazer, and wear three or four (or more!) skinny bangles. Opt for "layers" of necklaces too. Three lockets or charms, each on a longer chain, will add interest to a plain sweater. For a dramatic fashion statement, team a long gold-chain necklace with a long silver one, or an opera-length rope of pearls with a long gold chain filled with dazzling, sparkly stones.

Add-Ons That Add Up to a Great Look

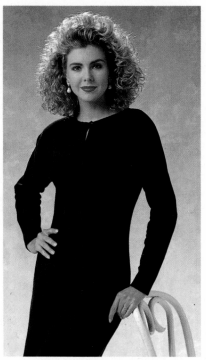

A plain black dress accessorized with a bold gold "collar" type necklace can add sparkle to your face.

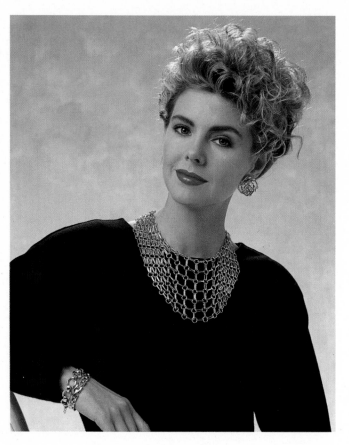

Here, a guide to the "cosmetic" side of accessories.

If your complexion or wardrobe is "cool," try earrings and necklaces in silver tones. Silver will catch, reflect light onto your face, brightening a pale or "tired" complexion. Other good bets: pearls with a blue-white or gray tone, faux ivory, plus "cool" stones like sapphires, garnets, lapis, onyx, opals, diamonds.

If your skin or clothing is "warm-toned," opt for gold accessories, earrings, and necklaces in shiny or matte finishes, to give your complexion glow. Other flattering choices: copper and brass pieces, plus creamy-colored or rosy pearls, "warm" stones like topaz, yellow-based jade, coral and turquoise, "yellow" diamonds.

· Give richness and warmth to olive skin with bronze-toned metals.

206

·Accent a tanned complexion with white or ivory jewelry.

·Warm up pale skin with red earrings, necklaces.

Love the look of black—but find that black sweaters, blouses, and jackets rob your face of color? A multi-strand pearl choker will warm your complexion. So will short, bold gold or silver necklaces (especially Egyptian "collar" types). Necklaces with brilliant mixes of multi-colored stones set in silver or gold, and faux ruby, emerald, topaz, or sapphire earrings rimmed in silver or gold, will catch—and play with—light around your face, adding sparkle.

If winter-white fashions leave you looking pale or sallow, wear earrings or a necklace combining gold with faux ivory, turquoise, or coral stones.

When choosing scarves, remember that lush, plush, or shiny fabrics will reflect light upward, onto the face (look for silk or silk-like materials with sheen). For evenings and holidays, opt for scarves with a hint of silver or gold woven throughout.

For evening, clip a dazzling rhinestone brooch (at least 3 by 3 inches) onto the neck of a black, red, purple, or other dramatically dark dress. The rhinestones will reflect a flattering light up under your chin and onto your face.

Choose jewelry to complement your hair color:

Hair	Jewelry
Brunette	Silver, pearls, burgundy, garnet
Gray	Silver and platinum
Auburn	Gold, amber, tiger's eye
Blonde	Gold, coral, pearls

Play up eye color with these beautiful choices:

Eyes	Jewelry
Blue	Sapphire, aquamarine, lapis
Green	Emerald, hazel tones, jade
Brown	Topaz, amber, tiger's eye, amethyst

Add-Ons That Add Up to a Great Look

FIT TO BE TIED

Create a wardrobe of scarves that suit your many moods, change your look from demure to dramatic in an instant. Want a classic look? Opt for a "signature silk," with an equestrian motif, or an interplay of gold coins and chains. Feeling romantic? Choose dusty floral prints or rich paisleys. Want to add a trendy twist to a simple dress or solid-color sweater and skirt duo? Look for tartan scarves in surprising colors like fuchsia (or scarves that *combine* tartan and floral motifs). Modern geometric designs and animal prints also add instant panache to more conservative clothes.

Be sure to buy scarves that flatter your outfit *and* your complexion:

- If your skin tone is *cool*, opt for scarves in solids or mixes of: black, stark white, soft and icy grays, deep navy, blue-red, purple, magenta, fuchsia, icy pink, raspberry, plum, mauve, burgundy, emerald green, and powder blue.

- If your complexion is *warm*, look for scarves in solids or mixes of: coffee, camel, honey, rust, beige, terra cotta, tomato red, creamy ivory, salmon, coral, gold, periwinkle blue, warm pastel pink, warm yellow, peach, buff, and clear navy.

ARTFUL ACCESSORIZING

Have fun when "styling" your outfit with accessories.

- Use pretty clip earrings (your mother's 1950's rhinestone pieces, or your own more modern clips) as pins. Fasten pairs onto the neckline of a plain jewel-neck sweater (keep them to one side, close to the shoulder).

- Combine the dazzling with everyday. Classic gold "Chanel" chains with distinctive pendants give "uptown" chic to a dressed-down denim jacket, white T, jeans, and "lizard" mocs.

Save time by coordinating jewelry to match your outfit the night before. In a rush? Keep a basic "accessory wardrobe" handy—a classic watch, a simple bracelet, a pair of hoop earrings— pieces that will go with almost any fashion look.

· Show off a slender waist by threading a colorful scarf through the belt loops on skirts, slacks, "Fred Astaire style."

· Tuck a lacy handkerchief into the pocket of a serious tailored blazer for an unexpected feminine touch.

· Wrap a rope of pearls around one wrist to create a "cuff."

Accessorize long hair with the following basics: several pairs of tortoise-shell barrettes or tortoise or black-enamel combs for day; a black satin or grosgrain bow or headband for a dressier evening look.

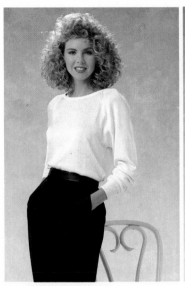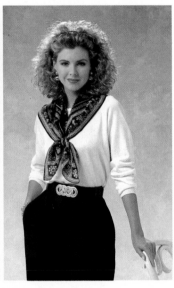

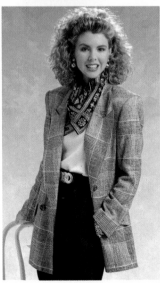

Use accessories to turn a basic outfit into a fashionable look, to take you from day to evening, and stretch your wardrobe options.

Add-Ons That Add Up to a Great Look

Great shoes, hosiery, and terrific handbags are important accessory items that can turn a plain outfit into a very special look. . . .

Simple pumps can be worn with most styles and can go from day to evening with the addition of clip-on shoe ornaments. Classic flats, loafers, and sandals are best for casual wear. Good leather shoes wear better and are better for your feet. Black, brown, and taupe are the most versatile colors.

Hosiery of different tones plays an important role in the ever-changing fashion scene. Sheer dark hose is best for those with very heavy legs. Thin legs? Try lacy or textured styles. Best to stay with natural, cream-toned sheers or barely black for work or day wear. For evening—or for the more adventuresome—fishnets, patterned hose, and brightly colored tights can be great add-ons to a wardrobe.

Classic-shaped handbags can take you from one season to the next. Buy the best handbag that you can afford—a good leather bag will last a longer time, especially if you tend to overstuff yours. A wardrobe of three handbags—an evening clutch, a dark leather, and a lighter-tone or patent purse—kept in proportion to your size, will finish any outfit no matter what your lifestyle.

If you are an eyeglass wearer, *keep in mind that they should work well with your choice of accessories. With larger frames or those that are bold in color, small earrings could get lost. If your frames are either silver or gold, you may wish to select coordinating jewelry pieces (see "Getting Framed," page 83).*

BEAUTY WRAP-UP

1. Use accessories—scarves, jewelry, belts—to transform a wardrobe of just a few basics into dozens of fashionable looks.

2. Select jewelry that's in proportion to your body size. If you're petite or small-boned, opt for smaller pieces that won't overwhelm you. Large-boned? Bigger, bolder earrings, necklaces, and scarves *won't* get lost on you.

3. Lengthen a petite figure, slenderize a rounder one, with oblong scarves, long ropes of pearls, or lengthy necklaces with pendants.

4. If you're thick- or short-waisted, choose skinny belts that don't cut you in half.

Real Beauty . . . Real Women

5. When wearing big, bold earrings, keep necklaces, pins, bracelets on the scaled-down side. If you go with a dramatic necklace or large pin, opt for smaller earrings.

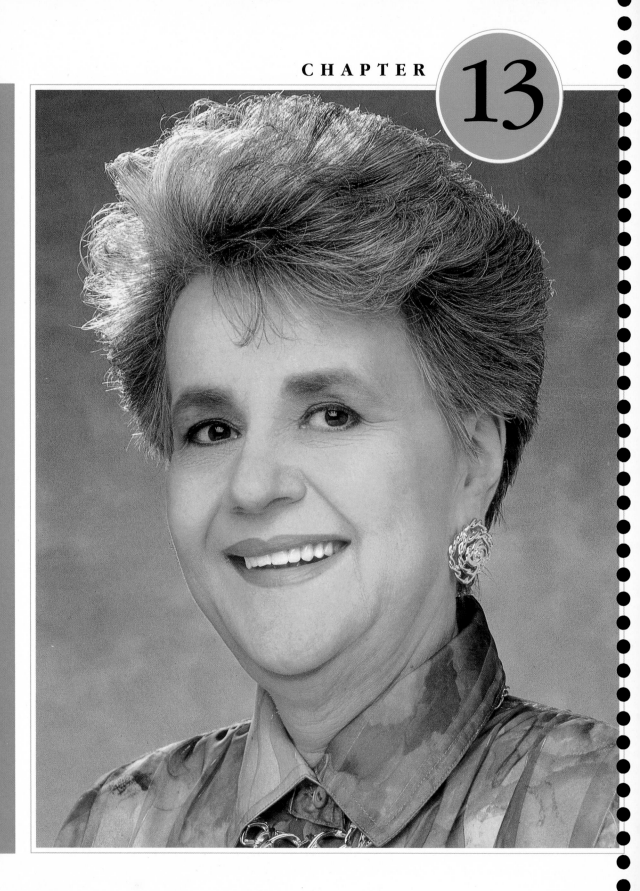

CHAPTER 13

From head to toe, you are constantly changing. Here's what to expect with the passing decades—and how you can look healthier, more beautiful, whether you're in your twenties or your sixties.

THE TWENTIES

Skin and Body. *What happens:* Your skin is at its best, rosy and healthy-looking (though too much time in the sun during your teen years may have caused some tiny premature wrinkling around the eyes, uneven skin texture and tone). By the mid-twenties, overly oily skin should calm down a bit. Your cheeks are plump, firm.

The twentysomething body is in peak condition, with limber muscles, strong bones.

What to do: Use gentle cleansers and moisturizers to keep skin in good condition. Wear sunscreen alone or choose a foundation or moisturizer containing sunscreen (and use an eye gel containing sunscreen, too, to protect against "crow's feet"). Choose sheer, water-based makeups. You can enjoy all cosmetic shades and forms. Don't overdo it, though, and be sure to thoroughly remove all makeup at the end of the day.

Don't take your physically fit body for granted. Eat a healthy diet and exercise daily. To ensure strong bones, include 1,200 mg. of calcium in your diet between the ages of twenty and twenty-four, at least 800 mg. from twenty-five to thirty (pregnant or breast-feeding women should add 400 mg. to the daily requirement). Menstruating women need 18 mg. of iron each day.

Hair. *What happens:* During the twenties, your hair is thick, luxurious (of course, over-zealous blow-drying, too-frequent perms, excessive highlight-

Looking Fabulous at Every Age

213

ing, straightening, and exposure to sun and chlorine *can* cause damage, dryness).

What to do: Wash hair daily with gentle shampoos and use light conditioners every day or every other day. Opt for subtle highlights, using products that contain little or no peroxide. Starting now, protect your hair from damaging UV rays by using styling products that contain sunscreen.

THE THIRTIES

Skin and Body. *What happens:* Thin, fine lines begin to appear around the eyes as oil glands slow production. Skin may become a bit drier and nails can start to peel, crack, or develop ridges. Your skin will also become a little sallow in your mid- to late thirties (the "rosy glow" of youth is gone), and your plumpish cheeks start to slim down as fat begins to redistribute itself. The skin begins to slacken slightly, as collagen breaks down. Tiny "broken" capillaries may appear around the nose, on the cheeks and chin (due to rosacea, heredity, or sun exposure), and "spider veins" crop up on legs. You may notice a few light age spots on your hands.

Generalized sagging begins body-wide (you may first notice a slightly "droopy" derrière). Breasts become a little less firm. Abdominal muscles tend to lose tone and firmness, especially if you've given birth. At thirty-five your bone density is at its peak.

What to do: Use moisturizing eye cream nightly, and an eye gel (with sunscreen) during the day to plump up fine lines. Step up moisturizer use on face and body, and, to restore rosy glow to the skin, try to get 25 minutes of aerobic exercise three to five times a week. Use collagen-boosting and moisturizing treatment products daily to slow down the appearance of aging. Pay special attention to the cheek area, where skin slackening shows up first. Minimize redness due to dilated capillaries by using a green or white makeup primer under foundation (or have them removed by a skilled dermatologist). Wear stockings with a little support to help prevent spider veins (a dermatologist can

214

inject veins with a special solution, causing them to collapse and "disappear").

If your skin is sallow, use a lavender under-makeup primer. Experiment with makeup; try different colors (always blend well and remember to coordinate shades with clothing and/or skin tone.)

Moisturize nails nightly with a rich cream, and use nail-strengthening enamels or ridge-filling base coat. Wear rubber gloves when doing dishes, and be sure to use a hand lotion containing sunscreen to prevent age spots. (Lighten age spots with o.t.c. skin-bleaching creams, or have a dermatologist lighten or remove them.)

Wear a bra that provides good support, and if you're into jogging, aerobics, or any other exercise that causes breasts to bounce, invest in a good sports bra to prevent stretching of, damage to, the connective tissues supporting the breasts. Be sure to include spot-toning exercises in your daily workout—abdominal crunches, upper body strengtheners, leg lifts. Keep bones strong by including 800 mg. of calcium in your diet daily (1,200 mg. if you're pregnant or lactating). Get an adequate amount of iron—18 mg.—from foods, or a multivitamin/mineral supplement.

Hair. *What happens:* As your oil glands gradually slow their output, your hair becomes a little drier. Coloring, straightening, perming—all can leave hair brittle, dull, if done too frequently or improperly. Hair also loses pigment in the thirties, and your color may look faded. Some gray hairs begin to appear.

What to do: Use a remoisturizing treatment once a week to restore shine, elasticity to hair. Rev up fading color with a gentle process, such as a vegetable glaze or a conditioning semi-permanent rinse (choose a shade that's close to your natural color), or put in subtle highlights in warm gold or red tones. Dry hair frequently gets "staticky." Curb flyaways by rubbing a dot of hairdressing into palms, then lightly running over hair. Go easy on gels, mousses, and sprays that contain lots of alcohol—they can rob hair of moisture and color. Choose products that *condition*.

Looking Fabulous at Every Age

THE FORTIES

Skin and Body. *What happens:* More fine lines show up around your eyes, and expression or "smile" lines start to appear around the mouth. The furrows running from the sides of your nostrils to the corners of your lips will become more pronounced. Your lips become thinner. Your skin may look dull, lackluster, flaky, due to increased dryness. Generalized sagging is more pronounced, and you may develop jowls or a little double chin. (African-American skin tends to age more gracefully than Caucasian complexions, and black women may not see these changes until their fifties.)

Body skin continues to slacken and you may notice a little flab or loose skin along the insides of upper arms. Breasts change shape, with the tops flattening out as gravity slowly distributes more tissue below the nipple.

What to do: Protect the delicate eye area with eye creams, and banish puffy lids, under-eye "bags" with cool compresses. Treat dry patches more frequently, opting for products containing retinol (vitamin A derivative) or glycolic acid, which penetrate into deeper layers of the skin. Facial moisturizers will plump up fine wrinkles, giving your skin a smoother, younger appearance. Exfoliate facial and body skin weekly to slough away dulling flakes. Stick with super-gentle cleansers and wash your face no more than twice daily (over-cleansing will emphasize fine lines). Use a richer makeup base (choose one with light moisturizing properties).

Use concealer pencil one or two shades lighter than your skin tone to "erase" deep furrows (smooth foundation over concealer). A dermatologist can fill in nose-to-mouth furrows with collagen injections, but this is a costly procedure that must be repeated several times a year (some women have reported allergic reactions to collagen injections).

There's no need to shy away from bright, clear makeup shades, but avoid iridescent colors—they'll emphasize wrinkles in the eye area. When choosing eyeshadows, avoid harsh colors or *bold* brights, which can "age" you. If you have pale eyes, flatter them with

216

makeup in rich browns, deep mauves. Dark eyes look beautiful in smoky grays, burgundies. Erase fine lines around lips with a lip fixative or toner. Choose a moisturizing lipstick in a light to medium tone (dark colors will make thin lips look almost nonexistent!). Use lip gloss to create the illusion of fuller lips.

To minimize droopy jowls, use foundation or a matte powder one shade darker than your usual color along jawline, blending well. To camouflage a double chin, smooth on foundation or powder one or two shades darker than usual makeup. Blend well with regular makeup.

Opt for soft, subtle blush in a matte formulation and translucent powder dusted *lightly* over skin.

Stick with your aerobic workouts and spot-toning exercises. Consider a simple weight-lifting program (many exercise tapes include techniques) to firm upper arms, strengthen muscles that support breasts.

Your diet should include 800 mg. of calcium and 18 mg. of iron each day.

Hair. *What happens:* Your hair is becoming increasingly dry—and a little coarse, due to slight graying (gray hair tends to be stiffer, more wiry than the rest of your hair). Many women complain of "dry scalp problems" (and related flakiness) as the oil glands on the scalp produce less lubrication. Your hair may look dull (particularly if you're a blonde or redhead) because the natural color is beginning to fade.

What to do: Brush hair nightly (about 15 strokes) to distribute oil down the length of hair. Use a remoisturizing shampoo and 60-second remoisturizing conditioner every day (you *may* want to cut back to every-other-day shampoos), and treat hair to a 10-minute deep conditioning treatment once a week.

To restore shine, use a leave-in protein conditioner (just a dab) on damp hair; protein coats the rough surface of dry hair, enabling it to catch and reflect light. Camouflage gray (and enrich your natural color) with a semi-permanent tint in a shade close to your natural hair hue, or opt for all-over highlights that mix several natural-looking shades to minimize gray (have a professional do the job for best results).

If your scalp's dry and flaky, once a week massage

217

with a remoisturizing conditioner (leave on for 5 minutes). A dandruff shampoo formulated for "dry scalp problems" will help reduce flaking.

THE FIFTIES

Skin and Body. *What happens:* Skin cells are turning over more slowly now, so your complexion (and body skin) looks dry, a little "powdery." Your skin will absorb makeup.

Eyelid droop is becoming more apparent. Age spots may appear on the face (they're also more pronounced on arms and backs of hands). All lines—around eyes, lips—and deep furrows along sides of nose, between brows, are more visible. Hands become wrinkled and small lines crop up on the chin.

If you're post-menopausal, you're at higher risk for bone loss, *and* for heart disease.

What to do: Continue your skin exfoliating regimen to slough away complexion-dulling flakes. Moisturize facial and body skin morning and night. If your skin is very dry, cleanse at bedtime only; in the morning, simply rinse with cool water. Consider having age spots on your face removed by a dermatologist; "erase" those on hands, arms with a skin-bleaching cream. Massage a rich moisture cream onto arms and hands several times daily to plump up wrinkles.

Avoid too-dark or overly bright nail colors like fire-engine red and burgundy, which can call attention to imperfect nails and wrinkles on hands. Instead, choose flattering shades of muted coral, soft pink, dusty rose.

Choose eye makeups that play down droopiness and puffiness. Opt for matte shadows in neutral tones like gray, taupe, mauve, and soft violet; sweep lightly starting at lashes and fading color toward brows. Moisturize area around your mouth to smooth out fine wrinkles. To keep lip color from feathering, line lips with a pencil that matches your lipstick. Use subtle powder blush (avoid frosteds) in rosy-peach, pinky-brown, or deeper shades of rose or dusty plum (steer clear of pale pink blush; it can leave skin looking pal-

218

lid). Opt for long-lasting moisturizing makeup in lieu of matte foundations, which can emphasize dryness. To keep makeup from fading, dust face lightly with translucent powder—but buff excess carefully; powder can accumulate in fine lines, emphasize wrinkles.

Continue your kind-to-skin-and-body aerobic and spot-toning exercises, and, to unkink muscles—which tend to tighten with age—do gentle stretches morning and night. Include 800 mg. of calcium per day in your diet (some experts recommend that women over fifty get 1,200 to 1,500 mg. a day) and 10 mg. of iron if you've stopped menstruating. Protect your heart with a heart-healthy diet (one that's low in sodium, cholesterol, and saturated fats) and have regular heart check-ups. If you're post-menopausal, ask your doctor about estrogen-replacement therapy, which may protect against heart disease and help prevent bone loss.

Hair. *What happens:* Many women notice general thinning of the hair during their fifties, initially in the temple and crown area, and possibly extending to the entire head. Your hair may simply look less full—or areas of your scalp may become visible. As your hair turns grayer, it will become coarser and drier. If you chemically process your hair, it can be brittle, fragile.

What to do: To give thinning hair an illusion of fullness, opt for body waves or curly perms (choose extremely gentle ones). Use mousse to "thicken" and texturize hair. (Some dermatologists are reporting success in reversing female-pattern baldness with the topical medication Rogaine, a form of the high-blood-pressure medicine minoxidil.)

Use a conditioning semi-permanent color to camouflage gray strands (choose one slightly lighter than your actual hair color; lighter colors are more flattering to over-fifty skin). Follow conditioning and deep-treatment regimens suggested in the "Forties" hair section, but try to shampoo every two or three days, if possible, to avoid over-drying your hair. If your hair needs to be styled daily (in between shampoos), just rinse with water, apply a super-light conditioner, rinse well, then blow-dry as usual.

THE SIXTIES AND BEYOND

Skin and Body. *What happens:* Fine lines are apparent on the cheeks. Crow's feet and wrinkles around the mouth are very pronounced. The cheeks start to become loose, droopy. You may develop hairs in the chin area, and hair may appear in the nostrils, around the nape of the neck. As you approach seventy, wrinkles (on your face, as well as arms and hands) may crease over each other, forming "nets." Your skin will be dry with a thin tissue-paper quality. More age spots will crop up on face, hands, and arms. Your neck may become "crepy," as will your eyelids.

You may shrink in height as bones become less dense.

What to do: Cleanse your face before bedtime to remove makeup; in the morning, rinse with clear, cool water. Apply a rich moisture cream to plump up wrinkles. Continue using retinol- and glycolic-acid–based beauty treatment creams in the evening. Opt for a sheer moisturizing foundation (a heavier one will look masky). Use eye cream at night, eye gel in the morning to "erase" wrinkles. Choose soft, subtle makeup shades (*avoid* "frosteds"); matte eyeshadows in neutral colors will minimize "crepy" quality of lids. A light sweep of moisturizing creamy blush in a medium-toned color will give your skin a healthy glow (avoid too-light shades, which will look fake, too-dark or too-bright ones, which can look clownish). Stroke a "stain" of natural-looking lip color over lips (be sure to "prime lips," prevent feathering, by using a lip toner first). If you use powder, choose for one with moisturizing ingredients—and use a super-light touch; too much powder will "sit" on your skin, looking "floury." As skin becomes drier and thinner, it can become increasingly sensitive: select hypoallergenic skin-care products and makeup.

Use small sharp scissors to clip hair in nostrils, and slant-edged tweezers to pluck chin hairs (you can also remove chin hair with a facial depilatory, but these products tend to irritate mature skin). Have a friend or your hairstylist shave the nape of your neck once a week or as needed.

Conceal a "crepy" neck with pretty scarves, stand-up collars, and turtleneck sweaters. Wear a longer-length necklace to detract from neck wrinkles.

Be sure to strengthen bones (and your heart!) with regular aerobic exercise (swim, walk briskly, or join a low-impact aerobics class). Include between 800 and 1,500 mg. of calcium in your diet daily, as well as 10 mg. of iron.

Hair. *What happens:* Your hair will turn predominantly gray—possibly white—as you near seventy (Asian and black women go gray a bit more slowly). Gray hair tends to be lackluster, dry, and unruly. It is also prone to "yellowness." You may find that your hair is quite thin and your scalp is visible.

What to do: Shampoo every three days or once a week, using a remoisturizing shampoo and 60-second remoisturizing conditioner. (If your hair is primarily gray, choose shampoos designed to take the yellow out, give hair a silvery hue.) Tame unruly hair with a once-a-week hot oil treatment.

To thicken hair, use mousse or hair-thickening products (look for mousse, gel, hairspray *formulated* for gray hair; regular products can trigger a yellowish cast). Or, create the illusion of fullness with a body wave or curly perm.

To cover gray, you'll need permanent hair color. (Choose a color one or two shades lighter than your natural color. If your hair *was* dark brown, select a medium-brown shade to give your complexion warmth.) Love the look of gray? Consider a shampoo-to-shampoo rinse designed to remove yellowish tinge, add luster, or a "gray optimizer," a semi-permanent color that gets rid of the yellow, brings out the silvery gloss in gray hair.

BEAUTY WRAP-UP

1. If you didn't use sunscreen religiously during your teen years to protect your skin against photoaging, *start in your twenties*. Smooth over skin *before* applying makeup.

2. Restore rosiness to thirtysomething skin by exercising aerobically. Be sure to "stockpile" calcium

(you need about 800 mg. daily) to prevent osteoporosis in later years.

3. In your forties, moisturize facial and body skin morning and night to prevent dryness, "plump up" fine lines. Exfoliate weekly to slough away skin-dulling flakes.

4. During the fifties, ask your doctor whether you should up your calcium intake to 1,200–1,500 mg. a day (post-menopausal women are at increased risk of bone loss). If your hair begins to thin, opt for a body wave or curly perm, or mousses or hair "thickeners" to create an illusion of fullness.

5. In your sixties, seventies and over, choose soft, subtle makeup shades (avoid frosteds, which can accentuate fine lines), and, if you decide to camouflage gray hair, choose a tint that's one or two shades lighter than your natural color (a dark shade can contrast too dramatically with mature skin and look artificial). Tame wiry or unruly gray hair with weekly conditioning treatments.

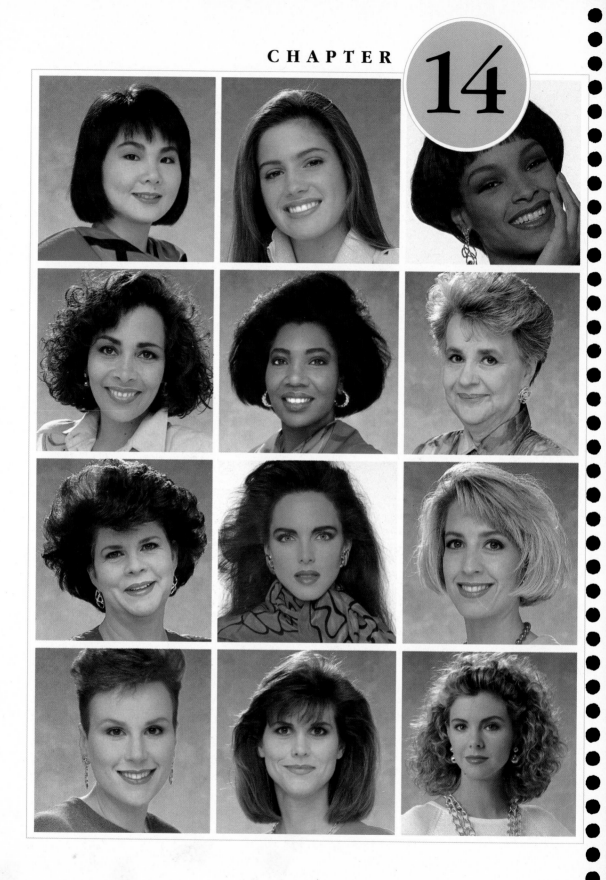

CHAPTER 14

JANUARY

If you're like most people, you fudged a bit (or a lot!) on your usually healthful diet over the holidays, and the pies, cakes, and cookies are beginning to show up on your tummy, hips, and thighs. Now's the time to seriously cut back on sweets and fats (limit yourself to a half cup of ice milk or low-fat frozen yogurt twice a week, or one small—but delicious—cookie every day). Snack on foods that satisfy your sweet tooth—sliced bananas with a pinch of sugar, a dash of cinnamon, and a topping of low-cal, no-fat, whipped-cream substitute, or a baked apple sweetened with fruit juice or sugar substitute, or rice cakes "frosted" with low-sugar fruit spread.

FEBRUARY

By now, winter temperatures—whether the bitter midwestern winds or the parching southwest sun—have taken a toll on your complexion, possibly leaving it dull and flaky. Treat yourself to a salon facial. Or, once a week pamper your skin with this "professional" facial—at home. Pour 1/4 cup chamomile flowers (available at drugstores) into 4 cups boiling water. Simmer 5 minutes. Pour water and flowers into a large bowl. Drape a towel over your head and steam your *clean* face for 5 minutes (hold face 8 inches from the bowl).

Beauty by the Month

Next, apply a skin-rejuvenating mask: Mix 2 tablespoons powdered brewer's yeast, 1 teaspoon apple juice, and 1 unbeaten egg white. Apply in a thick coating over your face and leave on for 10 to 15 minutes. Yeast blots up oil without stripping the skin of natural moisture. Egg white and apple juice act as mild astringents that texturize your complexion, leaving it smooth and silky.

MARCH

Your hair has succumbed to the winter doldrums. Restore shine and elasticity with a hot oil treatment. Heat 1/8 cup olive oil warm, not hot and massage through *dry* hair, from roots to ends. Wrap plastic wrap, then a large, warm towel around your head (heat towel in a hot dryer for 10 minutes to warm). Leave on for 30 minutes. Remove towel and wrap; massage shampoo directly onto hair—*then* add water to work up a lather. Rinse *well*. Your hair will look—and feel—like spun silk.

March is the ideal time to start your swimsuit shape-up. If you're 5 or 10 pounds over your perfect weight, begin cutting back on sweets, fats, and in-between-meal snacks. Aim to lose 1 to 2 pounds a week max. Start (or step up) an aerobic exercise program, walking, jogging, swimming, or biking at least 25 minutes daily, three to five times a week.

APRIL

Lighten up! As the weather turns warmer, put away your richer cleansers, moisturizers, and creamier makeups, switching to lighter products. Look for new makeup shades, too. Deeper, darker makeups will look too "heavy" during the spring. Choose lighter, brighter, clearer eyeshadow, blush, and lip colors.

Your hair color may be looking a little faded, due to the effects of damp or cold temperatures during the long winter. Add richness, brilliance to your hair with subtle golden or reddish highlights (choose gentle, at-home, semi-permanent color, or book a salon appointment for a vegetable glaze or highlighting).

MAY

If you haven't already switched to lighter, airier nail enamels, do so now. Select soft peaches, corals, honey-buffs, icy pinks, and soft violets. Get your feet ready for summer sandals—treat yourself to a salon pedicure, or do your own at home (every one to two weeks!).

Take advantage of spring evenings to get *outdoor* exercise (fresh air and aerobic workouts give your complexion a rosy, healthy glow). Intensify your sun-screen use, making sure you apply one that's suited to your skin type *under* foundation every morning. Slather onto arms, backs of hands—and neck, too.

JUNE

Experiment with various "self-tanning" lotions to find the one that works best on your particular skin type. Invest in "sun-kissed" makeups—bronzing pow-der, tawny blush; dust over cheeks, onto temples, across the bridge of your nose, and onto shoulders for a healthy glow.

If you swim, try to get in a few laps every day. Swimming provides one of the best cardiovascular workouts around (it's ideal for people with arthritis, since it puts less pressure on joints than any other ex-ercise).

Follow a warm-weather diet. Heavier meat dishes are hard to digest in hot weather. Switch to pasta sal-ads, fresh broiled fish, lots of fruit, and, for a midday pick-me-up, a fresh-fruit/protein shake you can whip up in your blender, pour into a thermos, and take to work: Combine 1 cup fresh raspberries or strawber-ries, 1/2 cup skim milk, 1/2 cup plain non-fat yogurt, 4 ice cubes, 1 tablespoon honey, 1 teaspoon vanilla fla-voring. Blend until thick and smooth. Makes 2 serv-ings.

JULY

Even if you've wisely protected your skin from the sun, by now your complexion's probably darkened at least a hint. Mix a slightly deeper foundation with your regular makeup to achieve a match close to your new skin tone.

Opt for opalescent or semi-frosted nail enamels in summery shades.

Use waterproof mascara (high temperatures, humidity, and perspiration can cause mascara to run).

If you swim frequently, use a shampoo designed to lift traces of potentially drying, damaging chlorine from your hair, and condition tresses daily.

AUGUST

As summer wanes, start an anti-blemish campaign (heat, humidity, the sun's rays, a tan—all can trigger breakouts). Exfoliate your complexion weekly to remove pore-clogging skin flakes, and before the first crop of pimples begins to appear, use a 2.5 percent benzoyl peroxide cream on oiliest areas every two or three days.

If you're ultra-prone to breakouts, schedule an appointment with your dermatologist *now*. Come September, his or her appointment calendar will be filled! (Ask for a skin cancer check, too.)

SEPTEMBER

As the weather starts to change, be aware of changes in your skin. Adapt your skin-care regimen accordingly, especially your moisturizing routine. If you use too-heavy moisturizers, or glop on lighter ones, you'll clog your pores. Smooth dry body skin with lukewarm hydrating baths: add a capful of your favorite bath oil to water, or 8 to 10 drops of any essential oil (rose, jasmine, lavender, eucalyptus).

Now is a good time to examine your nails and cuticles. If your cuticles are rough and dry, massage them every night with a rich cuticle cream or warmed olive or baby oil. Pay special attention to feet, too. Strappy sandals leave feet exposed, and your heels, bottoms of toes, may be rough and cracked. Use a pumice stone to rub away rough skin after every shower or bath, and massage feet with moisturizer.

OCTOBER

It's time to change makeup shades. Switch from lighter blush, eyeshadow, and lip colors to ones that are richer, deeper, more intense. For nails, choose creamy matte shades in berries, mauves, rich roses, wines, coffee, garnet.

If your hair's dried out, or a little brassy or reddish (due to too much time in the sun or in chlorinated water), deep condition weekly with a remoisturizing treatment. Massage into wet hair before you step into the shower or bath—let the heat and humidity "lock in" conditioner while you bathe. Tone down brassiness or redness with special color-correcting shampoos.

NOVEMBER

Get ready for the holidays by booking cut, color, or perm appointments for the *first* week of the month. From mid-November until January 1, your hair salon will be jam-packed. Luxurious highlights or glossy all-over, semi-permanent color will add richness, depth, and movement to your hair—and you'll feel (and look) especially pretty at holiday gatherings.

The pace is hectic this month, and you'll be busy juggling family responsibilities, career, parties, and holiday shopping. We all tend to get run down this time of year, so to protect yourself, consider getting a flu shot—and be sure to take a multivitamin every day to keep yourself in peak health. Eat smart, too, including an energy-boosting breakfast and lunch in your diet.

DECEMBER

Evoke the richness of the season by surrounding yourself with scent. Choose opulent perfumes and colognes, and retreat to a deliciously scented bath at least once a week (to rest and renew yourself in body and mind). Hang fragrant wreaths on inside doors, and place bowls of potpourri throughout the house.

Look for richness in cosmetics, too, and add a touch of glitter for special holiday evenings (holiday parties are the perfect time to experiment with brighter, bolder makeup looks; extravagant hair and fashions). Try a pearlized shadow swept over lids, a glimmering, "iced" lip color smoothed onto lips, or opalescent nail enamel slicked over a creamy color.

Holidays prompt nonstop nibbling. Curb your appetite by eating a sensible dinner before heading out to a party. Once you arrive, snack on crudités (but skip the dip). Opt for seltzer with a twist of lime (it's filling!) in lieu of fattening eggnog or other alcoholic beverages.

Above all, celebrate the beauty of the season—and *yourself.*

Real Beauty . . . Real Women

About the Author

Kathleen Walas, Avon's International Beauty and Fashion Director, has been in the beauty and fashion business for over 15 years. She is co-author of the bestseller *Taking Control of Your Life: The Secrets of Successful Enterprising Women* and travels extensively throughout the United States and overseas as a cosmetics and appearance expert, teaching consumers how to adapt current beauty and fashion trends to their own lifestyles.

Ms. Walas has shared her tips on developing personal style with millions through television, radio, and newspaper interviews. Her beauty hints and makeovers have been featured in such publications as *Woman's Day*, *McCall's*, *Harper's Bazaar*, *Ladies' Home Journal*, *New Woman*, and *Cosmopolitan*.

Before joining Avon, she was a consultant to dozens of actresses, models, and fashion designers, including Faye Dunaway, Mary Tyler Moore, Lauren Hutton, Dorothy Hamill, Jill Clayburgh, Kim Alexis, and Adrienne Vittadini.

Wife, mother of two sons, and co-owner of a flourishing beauty-care business, Ms. Walas is a terrific role model for the nineties.

Additional copies of *Real Beauty . . . Real Women* may be ordered by sending a check for $19.50 (please add the following for postage and handling: $2.00 for the first copy, $1.00 for each added copy) to:

MasterMedia Limited
17 East 89th Street
New York, NY 10128
(212) 260-5600
(800) 334-8232
fax: (212) 348-2020

Kathleen Walas is available for speeches and workshops. Please contact MasterMedia's Speakers' Bureau for availability and fee arrangements. Call Tony Colao at (908) 359-1612; fax: (908) 359-1647.

Index

Favorite Beauty Tips from Avon Representatives Across the Country

Be as healthy as possible—get plenty of sleep and exercise; maintain a balanced diet; wear colors and styles that reflect your personality; have a positive attitude. When you feel good, you look good!

June Griggs, N. Charleston, SC

An effective skin-care program must be followed everyday without fail. My skin-care program includes drinking at least one quart of water a day, plus sleeping on a satin pillow case or on my back to prevent sleep wrinkles.

Dorothy Chavers, Andalusia, AL

Start using Avon skin-care products at an early age, morning and night, especially eyecare products. Keep them in the refrigerator to give the area around your eyes a quick cool lift. Wear sunglasses outside . . . no squinting!

Naomi Hills, Martinsville, IL

Regular washcloths can be too abrasive to some facial skin. When washing your face, apply your favorite cleanser and use a baby washcloth! Great for sensitive skin.

Margaret Hunsinger, Elysburg, PA

I apply Pore Reducer Beauty Treatment, place cucumber slices over each eye, recline, sip an 8 oz. glass of lemon water, and listen to Mozart for 15 minutes. I get that healthy, glowing look; am refreshed and relaxed. What a beauty boost!

Lora Black, Lincoln, NE

Give your scalp a massage when you shampoo. Press the flat of your fingertips on your scalp and rub with circular motions, from side to side (feel your scalp move). Watch how your hair glows after a few treatments.

Vicki Ryan, Winter Haven, FL

When too much summer fun in the pool leaves your hair with that "green" tint—bring out the tomato juice! Saturate hair with the juice, leave on for 15 minutes, and then wash and condition hair with your favorite Avon hair products. Out with the "green"—in with the "sheen"!

Marie Mashburn, Calhoun, GA

Put lotion on your hands before you put on gloves to wash dishes or do chores. Your hands will be really super-soft when you're done!

Diane Padelford, Bradenton, FL

Making up a face is comparable to artwork. You can't paint a perfect picture on a dirty canvas! For your perfect look, start with a clean face.

Jodie Hetherington, Gladwin, MI

Want your makeup to look fresh longer? Cleanse, tone and moisturize as usual, then rub an ice cube across face (or use ice wrapped in a towel) before applying makeup. Lines and puffiness will seem to disappear; makeup goes on easier, stays fresh longer, and you'll feel fresh and rejuvenated.

Martha Love, Spring Valley, CA and
Barbara J. Martin, Fair Lawn, NJ

When applying eye concealer, it's important to apply little pressure around the eye area (to prevent premature wrinkling). By using the tip of your ring finger, the amount of stress applied is minimal.

Bonnie Morice, Glendale, AR

When applying eyeliner, eyeshadow, mascara or whatever eye makeup you use, NEVER pull your eyelid back tight. You may be tempted to do so to get a straight line, but eventually you will have created lines or wrinkles!

Marie Nelson, Phoenix, AR

Smile BIG when applying blush. This outlines the apple of the cheek where color should be applied and will keep the blush out of the creases around the eyes, nose and mouth.

Jean Long, Kokomo, IN

Before putting eyeshadow on, I apply a small amount of oil-control powder on the eyelids. This keeps the eyeshadow from creasing and keeps them fresh-looking all day.

Sandra Clow, Chicopee, MA

Caught without a tissue to blot your lipstick? Simply form a circle with your lips, in an "O" shape, insert your index finger in halfway and pullout. Any lipstick that would have stuck to your teeth is now on your finger. (Wipe your finger with the other hand and it's gone.)

Trish Arnold, Mt. Vernon, WA and
Elaine S. Taillac, San Diego, CA

For women who work under fluorescent lights . . . wear matte makeup rather than frosts. Frosts tend to reflect light and make you look washed out or shiny while matte products have a smoother appearance and look more professional.

Colelyn S. Blakely, Salt Lake City, UT

Always store mascara tubes upside down. The mascara drains down to the neck and coats the brush everytime it's pulled out. This eliminates pumping and scraping to try to get mascara on the brush!

Leslie Ann Crevier, St. James, MN

When using the powder puff of pressed powder compacts, store the puff in the compact with the fluffy side up. The oil from wiping your face will not absorb into the pressed powder and your compact lasts much longer.

Marlys Monahan, Waseca, MN

Pulling together a "look" in the morning can be chancy as we rush to beat the clock. I lay out my outfit the night before, down to earrings and lipstick color. Hardly a day passes that I do not receive a compliment, making my hectic day more pleasant!

Susan Ani, Wilmette, IL

I utilize old standbys to create new fashion accessories. One favorite is braiding beads into a scarf to give my wardrobe — and me — a new look. When I look good, I feel great!

Barbara Hocking, Lombard, IL

Dress and act as if this is your most successful day. Feel good about yourself!

Amy C. Eversole, Delsware, OH

And from all of our Avon Representatives: The most popular and best beauty tip of all is SMILE—you'll look better, feel better, and it's free!

If you would like more information on ordering Avon Products, call 1 (800) 858-8000.

Avon Skin Care

FACIAL

DAILY REVIVAL
   Everyday necessities for healthy looking skin.

1. *Dry Skin*
   • Gentle Cream Cleanser
   • Super Moisture Cream
2. *Normal/Combination Skin*
   • Mild Cleansing Bar
   • Foaming Facial Wash
   • Softening Toner
   • Active Moisture Lotion with Paba-Free Sunscreen
3. *Oily Skin*
   • Oil Balancing Bar
   • Oil Clearing Wash
   • Conditioning Pore Refiner
   • Oil-Free Moisture Factor
4. *For All Skin Types*
   • Fragrance-Free Moisture Lotion for Super-Sensitive Skin
   • Eye Lift Creme
   • Night Cream

AVON ADVANCED BEAUTY TREATMENTS
   Our most effective skin care to help minimize the signs of time.

1. BioAdvance
   For early signs of aging; helps improve the appearance of fine dry lines.
2. BioAdvance 2000
   For older-looking skin; helps target the signs of facial aging of older skin.
3. Anew Perfecting Complex for Face
   Helps achieve and restore healthy looking skin.
4. Collagen Booster
   Maintains younger looking skin.
5. Advanced Night Support
   Skin revitalizing formula; counteracts environmental damage while you sleep.
6. Moisture Shield
   With SPF 15; protects from UV damage.
7. Tinted Moisture Shield
   With SPF 15; protects from UV damage (with natural face tint).

8. Nutura Replenishing Creme
   Extra moisturization.

AVON VISIBLE IMPROVEMENT PROGRAM
   Modern solutions to special problems.

1. Maximum Moisture
   Super hydrating complex
2. Eye Perfector
   With liposomes
3. Blemish Solver
   Medicated touch stick
4. Visible Advantage
   Skin reviving liquid
5. Skin Refiner
   Gentle action scrub
6. Spotlite Banishing Stick
   Skin lightener with sunscreen
7. Banishing Cream
   Skin lightener with sunscreen
8. Shine Solution
   8-hour oil controlling liquid
9. Dramatic Firming Cream
   For face and throat
10. Pore Reducer
   Beauty treatment mask
11. Cellulite Contour
   Beauty treatment

CLEARSKIN
   That's a promise!

1. Antibacterial Cleansing Scrub
2. Antibacterial Cleansing Cake
3. Antibacterial Astringent Cleansing Lotion
4. Maximum Strength Cleansing Pads
5. Clarifying Mask
6. 10% Benzoyl Peroxide Cream

HAND AND BODY

MOISTURE THERAPY
   Starts to heal and comfort extremely dry skin on contact.

1. Body Lotion 14 oz.
2. Body Lotion 7 oz.
3. Bath Oil 14 oz.

4. Hand Cream 4.5 oz.
5. Extra Strength Cream 6 oz.
6. Body Cleanser
7. Liquid Soap
8. Hand Cream with SPF-8 2.25 oz.
9. Shampoo

RICH MOISTURE
Helps maintain skin's natural moisture balance for beautiful skin.

1. Body Lotion 16 oz.
2. Hand/Nail Cream 4.5 oz.
3. Face Cream 7 oz.
4. Face Cream 3.5 oz.
5. Rich Moisture Water Rinseable Cold Cream 3 oz.

CARE DEEPLY
Don't just care for your family's skin . . .
CARE DEEPLY.

1. Body Lotion 10 oz.
2. Hand Lotion 4.5 oz.
3. Lip Balm .15 oz.

SILICONE GLOVE
Lasting protection for hard-working hands.

1. Hand Cream 4.5 oz.
2. Hand Cream 2.25 oz.

AVON ESSENTIALS
Derived from nature to nourish your skin.

1. Skin Balancing Lotion
2. Milky Cream Facial Cleanser
3. Soothing Hand and Body Lotion
4. Gentle Body Polisher
5. Invigorating Shower Gel

VITA MOIST
Vitamin enriched to help keep skin soft, smooth and supple.

1. Body Lotion 16 oz.
2. Hand/Nail Cream 4.5 oz.
3. Hand/Nail Cream 2.25 oz.
4. Face Cream 7 oz.
5. Face Cream 3.5 oz.
6. Foam Bath 8 oz.

Avon Color

LIPS

Color Rich Lipstick—Creamy, full coverage enriched with lip-smoothing moisturizers.

Satin Smooth Lipstick—Light, silky lipstick with moisturizers to keep lips soft and kissable.

Color Release Lipstick—Long-wearing, this creamy vibrant full-coverage lipstick releases fresh color throughout the day.

Crystal Shine Gloss Stick—Sheer, shining color formulated to moisturize and help protect.

Luxury Lip Lining Pencil—Lines and defines lips; luxurious pencil glides on even, long-wearing color.

Luxury Lip Coloring Pencil—Glossy, long–lasting color with luscious shine in a pencil.

Glimmerstick Lip Lining—Self-sharpening, creamy lip liner.

Glimmerstick Lip Coloring—Wide color in a pencil with a swivel-up tip that never needs a sharpener.

Unlimited Moisture Lipstick—Continually moisturizes and conditions. True color pay-off with SPF 15.

EYES

Silk Finish Eyeshadows—Silky powders enriched with encapsulated moisturizers for extra creaminess; apply smoothly and blend beautifully. Long wearing and color-true all day.

Single
Duo—2 coordinated colors
Quad—4 coordinated colors

Luxury Eye-Lining Pencil—Lines and defines, long-lasting, waterproof.

Luxury Eye-Coloring Pencil—Soft and blendable, glides on effortlessly, waterproof, crease resistant.

Glimmerstick Eye Lining—A sleek pencil with a twist-up tip; glides on smooth, blendable color. Self-sharpening.

Glimmerstick Eye Coloring—Creamy, blendable color; all the ease of coloring pencil with no sharpener needed.

Glimmerstick for Brows—Natural brow color; soft and blendable in a swivel-up, self-sharpening tip.

Color Glide Liquid Eyeliner—Line and define eyes with vibrant and lustrous long-lasting color. Natural-bristle brush.

MASCARA

Lots O'Lash—Thickens.

Body Workout—Body building, conditions.

Pure Care—For contact lens wearers.

Wash-Off Waterproof—Washes off with soap and water.

Advanced Waterproof—Wears for 24 hours.

Model Perfect—Colors and curls.

BLUSH

Natural Radiance Single—Smooth and long-wearing. Brush-on natural glow.

Color Release Long-Wearing Blush—Color renews itself and outwears any other blush: it looks just-put-on for so much longer.

Natural Radiance Blush Stick—Creamy, moisturizing, blendable color in a swivel-up case. So easy to use.

FACE: FOUNDATIONS

1. *Enhancing Liquid*—For normal to dry skin, medium coverage. Contains a balancing-moisturizing system for natural looking finish.

2. *Oil-Free Liquid*—Normal to oily skin, light coverage. Controls oiliness and shine without depriving skin of natural moisture. Water-based with a matte finish.

3. *Pure Care Gentle Liquid*—For sensitive skin, gentle and fragrance-free, medium to light coverage. Moisturizes skin while keeping it looking natural and fresh.

4. *Perfecting Creme*—For dry to very dry skin, medium-plus coverage. Rich moisturizing, souffle-like formula leaves skin looking smooth, even, flawless.

5. *Natural Finish Creme Powder*—For oily skin, medium to light coverage. Sponges on like a cream but dries to a silky powder finish.

CONCEALERS

1. *Concealing Stick*—Medium coverage; covers imperfections while it helps moisturize.
2. *Pure Care Concealer*—The gentle perfector; lightweight, creamy formula provides natural looking coverage of flaws and helps soften lines around eyes.
3. *Hide N' Blend Body Cover*—Full coverage. Covers stretch marks, blemishes and bruises. Helps conceal veins, birthmarks and scars. Waterproof.
4. *Next Generation Concealer*—To be introduced late in 1992.

POWDERS

1. *Translucent Face Powder*—Pressed, light-reflecting for an ultra-smooth look that lasts for hours; portable.
2. *Translucent Face Powder*—Loose, natural-bristle brush smooths on powder easily for a sheer, natural look.
3. *Oil Control Powder*—Pressed, helps control shine. Oil breakthrough is controlled for up to 8 hours as it evens out skin tone for a soft, matte finish.
4. *Pressed Bronzing Powder*—Gives your skin the natural glow and shimmer of a radiant suntan.

NAIL CARE

1. *Maximum Length Nail Program*—Focused nail treatment that protects and seals the nail surface for stronger, longer, more beautiful nails.
2. *Hydra-Moist Nail Conditioning Pearls*—Unique, encapsulated gel restores natural moisture to nails. Contains precious pearls of a specially-blended hydrating complex.
3. *Always Smooth Cuticle Conditioner*—Softens and moisturizes dry cuticles. Wand applicator gently pushes back cuticles.
4. *Mira Cuticle Vanishing Complex*—Ragged edges of cuticles vanish within 14 days. Eliminates hard cuticule build-up, giving that just-manicured look.
5. *Ridge-Free Base Coat*—Provides the perfect surface for smooth, even nail-enamel application.
6. *No-Peel Smoother*—Base coat for peeling, layered nails. Helps nails resist peeling.
7. *Ultra Hard Strengthener*—Base coat for soft, thin, weak nails. Provides hardener to make nails firmer and stronger. Protects against bending.
8. *No-Split Bonder*—Base coat for dry, brittle nails that break easily. Helps prevent splitting, cracking, and breaking.
9. *No Chip Top Coat*—Protects polish from chipping and gives nails a high lustre.

DISCRETES

1. Flavor Saver Lip Balm
2. Slick Tints
3. Dew Kiss
4. Fine Line Eye Pen
5. Single Stroke Nail Enamel
6. Quick Change Nail Color
7. Effective Eye Makeup Remover
8. Pure Care Eye Makeup Remover

Personal Beauty Notes